THE
HEALER
WITHIN

Lisa /

The mystery of Self Healing
is no mystery.

Roger Jahnke

THE
HEALER
WITHIN

O

The Four Essential Self-Care
Methods for Creating
Optimal Health

Roger Jahnke,
Doctor of Oriental Medicine

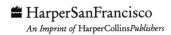
HarperSanFrancisco
An Imprint of HarperCollins*Publishers*

[🌲] A TREE CLAUSE BOOK

HarperSanFrancisco and the author, in association with The
Basic Foundation, a not-for-profit organization whose primary
mission is reforestation, will facilitate the planting of two trees
for every one tree used in the manufacture of this book.

HarperCollins Web Site: http://www.harpercollins.com

HarperCollins®, [📖] ®, and HarperSanFrancisco™ are
trademarks of HarperCollins Publishers Inc.

Illustrations by Karen Kuchar. Special thanks to Eben G.
Jahnke for the hand, foot, and ear charts and the massaging
hands positions in the massage chapter.

FIRST EDITION

Library of Congress Cataloging-in-Publication Data

Jahnke, Roger.
    The healer within : the four essential self-care methods
  for creating optimal health / Roger Jahnke.
    Includes bibliographical references and index.
    ISBN 0–06–251476–8 (cloth)
    ISBN 0–06–251477–6 (pbk.)
    1. Self-care, Health. 2. Alternative medicine. 3. Healing.
  I. Title.
RA776.95.J34   1997
615.5—dc21   96–38129

97 98 99 00 01 ❖ RRD(H) 10 9 8 7 6 5 4 3 2 1

○

To every individual who takes self-healing action. You are helping the human race to remember how to awaken and master the healer within. To the parents, grandparents, teachers, neighbors, and friends who pass this practical wisdom on to the children.

To the health care organizations, physicians, nurses, health educators, and wellness professionals who are actively implementing programming founded on health enhancement, stress mastery, and the interactions of the body, mind, and spirit. To teachers, politicians, corporate executives, ministers, and rabbis who encourage health enhancement. As you offer this knowledge and these tools to the people in your community, you are demonstrating service and love of the highest order. You are fostering the return of the lost value of self-reliance, so critically needed in our communities today.

To my circle of mentors, which includes numerous ancient and modern physicians, Native American medicine people, Chinese and Ayurvedic doctors, Hawaiian healers, and especially my own grandmother, who taught me self-healing methods in my youth.

To Marjorie Love, who administered liberal doses of love and support, the profound medicines that mothers give. She was able to offer me the freedom to follow my own alternative impulses, which have now led to this remarkable work in the realm of human empowerment through practical wisdom and inspiration.

And to Rebecca, from a heavenly source, a co-worker in life's fascinating flow, who heals through the sound of her voice, her listening, and her connection to the divine.

Contents

Acknowledgments

My grateful acknowledgment for your support and encouragement is most sincere.

In the world of books: Andrew Weil for pointing out a way in what seemed like impassable complexity. Jeremy Tarcher for patient guidance, clear and benevolent. Larry Dossey for his pure ideals and his kind support, and for helping to shine the light of science on the human spirit. Muriel Nellis, my agent, for opening a door where none could be seen. Caroline Pincus, my editor, for gentle brilliance—an artist in the human realm as well as in literature. Now I know why authors adore their editors. The Harper San Francisco team—Paul, Sally, Amy, Greg, Rosana—practical, tireless, spirited.

In the realm of health enhancement, the self-healing arts, and medicine: To Taoist Master Chang Yi Hsiang (Dr. Lily Siou), who gave me entry into the beautiful mystery of Chinese Taoist Medicine and revealed Qigong (Chi Kung) as the source, heart, and essence of the Asian healing arts. To Weng Chi-Hsiu (Daniel Weng), who taught me the value of dedicated training in Kungfu through his own discipline and who gave me my first and favorite Taiji (Tai Chi). To Doctor Ernest Shearer, who transformed me from a student of medicine into a clinician with a powerful vision of the healer within. To the wonderful, open-hearted master teachers at the institutes, hospitals, and temples in China who have so freely shared the arts of self-healing with a hope for worldwide healing. To the members of the original Wednesday Practice Session, who helped to bring the health enhancement methods to a broader audience, and to the hospitals in Santa Barbara as well as the Adult Education program and the City Recreation program for helping to support the weekly practice session over the years.

Declaration of Health Independence

When the people are even mildly enlightened,
oppression of the body and mind will disappear.

Thomas Jefferson,
farmer, philosopher, social architect

Thomas Jefferson, the greatest revolutionary thinker in American history and the author of the Declaration of Independence, also wrote an innovative book on health self-reliance that urged people to free themselves from the need for medicine and doctors whenever possible. His close friend Benjamin Rush, who was a cosigner of the Declaration of Independence and the personal physician to George Washington, wrote, "The Constitution of this new republic must make special privilege for medical freedom as well as religious freedom." Both of these great thinkers agreed that citizens must have the right and the responsibility to protect and enhance their own health and vitality in order to build and sustain the new nation.

Through the American Revolution, people rejected the tax on tea, eliminated their dependence on England and the king, and claimed their spiritual freedom. Now many Americans are feeling a new revolutionary urge to reduce their dependence on the health care system, cut the cost of medicine, and achieve health self-reliance.

A great economic tide has shifted throughout the world. Once wealthy nations, the United States and other countries in the Western world are now terribly challenged economically. A major culprit in this indebtedness is the high cost of health care and a system that has created nationwide dependence on medical providers. Dozens of strategies have failed to heal this wound in health care. Until recently little was done to remind people that they can often avoid medical visits simply by engaging in health

enhancement and disease prevention practices. As we will discuss, Americans have the potential to save over half of what they
spend every year on health care!

Every governmental body—from community leaders, to state
governments, to nations, and even to the World Health Organization—has called for a concerted effort to protect and enhance
health. However, governments seem trapped in their struggles for
power, and the medical system is generally still focused on disease, rather than health. The insurance industry is really just that:
an industry. Its product is, unfortunately, not health. People, it
seems, will have to resolve this crisis on their own.

Transforming the health care system would seem an insur-
mountable task if it were not for one astounding fact: we produce
within us a remarkable natural healing resource. It is the "healer
within." The human body comes with its own standard equipment
for self-healing. Powerful yet simple self-healing methods will create a critically needed revolution in health care and medicine.

Genuine health care, because of the nature of the healer
within, creates health independence. And such a rebirth of self-
reliance is desperately needed, not only in America but throughout the world. Our knowledge of the healer within gives us the
ability to declare our independence.

All the necessary biological components of self-healing have
been in place for thousands of years. Both ancient and contemporary philosophers have pointed to it. Science has now confirmed
it. (Simple discussion of the physiology of the healer within will
accompany the practices in part 2. A more detailed discussion is
in the appendix.) The most profound healer is within us—we
produce our own internal medicine. It is easy to turn this medicine on. And it is absolutely free.

Learning and doing the self-applied health enhancement
methods in the final years of the twentieth century may be as pa-
triotic as joining America's revolutionary army under General
Washington in 1776, as following Joan of Arc in the French battle
against the English in the fifteenth century, or as walking across
India with Mahatma Gandhi in the 1940s. A multitude of self-
reliant and healthy people creates a powerful force for change.

Entire communities have already begun to see the value of
community-wide health enhancement. Dozens of communities

throughout the United States, Europe, and Canada have made it their goal to become the "healthiest community" or the "wellness capital" in their region. In Europe the "Healthy Cities" movement is supported by the World Health Organization. In the United States one of the most important annual meetings of hospitals and health care providers is called the "Healthy Communities Summit."

Corporations and hospitals have already begun to encourage health independence strategies in order to increase productivity and improve the health of their communities. Teachers will be able to use this knowledge to encourage health self-reliance in our children, and physicians will be able to give this knowledge to their patients. Grandmothers will teach health secrets to their grandchildren again, as grandmothers have done throughout most of human history.

We each have the opportunity to participate as an independent agent in a dramatic transformation of human culture. Crime, poverty, environmental pollution, drug and alcohol addiction, and many other problems beg for a renewal of informed individualism and the pioneer spirit. For anyone, taking on these challenges seems immense, even impossible. But the first step toward improving the world is actually quite reasonable: simply, independently, and calmly improve yourself!

When people learn about the healer within themselves and then take action to care for their own physical, mental, emotional, and spiritual health, they are transformed. Victims of life's problems become independent and empowered creators of better health, greater joy, and positive living. Instead of handing over the power to others, they retain the authority to make their own choices and to participate in an exciting era of change. Self-directed citizens are powerful leaders and role models for their children, grandchildren, and fellow community members.

You personally have only one responsibility. Simply apply the practices yourself. If you wish, share them with others. Your daily practice alone makes you a part of the solution by reducing the likelihood that you are a part of the problem. You become a participant in an exciting revolution. And as an added benefit, you will become a healthier, more productive, and more energetic person.

Making a Miracle

Patricia remembers freezing rain quickly transforming the road-way into ice, her surprise as she felt her car suddenly spinning out of control, and the terrifying sound of shattering glass. Then, after an indefinite period of unconsciousness, she heard the soothing voice of a deer hunter: "I'm an off-duty emergency medical technician. You are in good hands, a hospital is nearby. We've already called for an ambulance. Please do not move or talk; you have been seriously injured." Patricia had been thrown from the car, and it had actually rolled over her. As she became aware that she was lying in a dark, ice-covered field, she realized that she was completely numb.

The ambulance rushed Patricia, in severe shock, to a local hospital. She remembers wiggling her toes and checking for teeth with her tongue. She felt really cold, and all she wanted to do was sleep. Her body was in severe pain; it would be a relief to rest. But she kept hearing the voice of the emergency medical technician: "Patricia, do not fall asleep!"

The little rural hospital nearby could not treat her complex injuries, so she was moved by another ambulance to a large medical center. Every few miles the driver stopped so that technicians could monitor her vital signs carefully. At the medical center she was listed in critical condition. A lung was punctured; it was nearly impossible for her to breathe. The CAT scan found that her liver was terribly bruised. Her spleen was seriously torn, nearly ruptured. She was bleeding internally from numerous injuries.

The physician team was prepared to rush her into emergency surgery to remove the damaged spleen. However, her situation was so serious that it was dangerous to operate before she had stabilized. The physicians wanted their work to improve her chances to live, not provide additional trauma. She could not receive pain medication, the doctor said, because it might diminish her body's ability to recover stability for the surgery.

So Patricia, in severe pain and with no medication, was told to hold on while the medical team waited to see if she would stabilize enough to be operated on. She had lost a lot of blood. Lying there in the intensive care unit, Patricia was suspended between living and dying. Ironically, she was in too critical a condition to receive pain-relieving medicine but not well enough to have life-saving surgery.

Patricia decided she wouldn't just wait. She was going in and out of consciousness, experiencing tremendous pain, and nearly unable to speak. But she was also in a state of heightened awareness. She decided to take personal action to ensure that the doctors would be able to operate and help her recover. "What can I do while I am in critical condition?" she wondered. Within her line of sight was a small ball in a clear glass tube that she could see rising and falling as her breath entered and exited her lungs. With each inhalation the ball would rise about a third of the way up the tube.

She remembered that the breath was mentioned again and again in the Bible. God created the world by releasing a breath on the vast waters. Life was given to the first human through sharing God's breath. The great psalm said, "Each life is but a breath." And Jesus purposefully put breath back into Lazarus and raised him up from death. Patricia's lung was punctured, and it was very difficult and painful for her to breathe at all. But she also remembered that Jesus said, "Your faith has healed you." So she took on the greatest challenge of her twenty-six years: to save her own life.

She decided to use her breathing and to rest in her faith. Over and over for hours, she struggled to breathe in. Then with each exhalation, she relaxed, resting in her faith. Every few moments she would deepen her inhalation just a tiny bit. It was painful, but she remembers being aware of a sense of improvement. With each exhalation she felt a wave of warmth throughout her body. Watching the little ball rise higher and higher was a kind of biofeedback; it confirmed that she was improving her situation.

She remembers looking at the clock at 2:15 A.M., almost eight hours after the crash. Just at that moment she was able to achieve her first full breath. She felt clear at that point that she had stabilized her condition so that the life-saving surgery would be possible. Even now, over a decade later, that moment stands out in her mind as lucid and connected to her deepest self—a turning point in her life.

In the morning the doctors reported that she had done astonishingly well and that she was stable enough to survive the operation. But they decided to keep her under observation a little longer before removing the spleen. Patricia continued her practice, deepening the breaths, deeply relaxing, and celebrating the promise that faith had healing power. Eventually, the doctors did an ultrasound diagnosis as preparation for the surgery. They discovered that both the liver and the torn spleen had miraculously repaired during the night! They decided that they did not need to remove the spleen at all.

The profound power of Patricia's story is that she was able to discover spontaneously her own self-healing ability. Her faith that she could heal, accompanied by the simple acts of deepening her relaxation and focusing on the breath, produced an extraordinary result. Without any special training, she made this breakthrough discovery on her own. Neither surgical procedures nor medications produced this healing, even though a team of highly skilled medical experts felt that surgery would be necessary to save her life. With the conscious use of the breath, relaxation, and the belief that she could help heal herself, she created what easily qualifies as a miracle.

Her spleen healed completely with no surgical or medical support, as did her punctured lung and severely bruised liver. On follow-up visits Patricia's physician expressed astonishment at her recovery. This young woman, so severely and traumatically injured in what appeared to be a fatal car crash, had literally called herself back from the brink of death.

Patricia's story is a celebration of two dramatic ideas that you are about to explore. First, there is a profound medicine, a powerful healing resource, produced naturally within us—this is the healer within. Second, through purposeful relaxation and regulation of our breath (and other simple self-healing methods including self-massage and gentle movement of the body), we can turn this medicine on.

A Bold Purpose

This book is intended to incite a revolution. When we learn to heal ourselves by activating our own internal medicine, we will be able to increase our productivity, our vitality, and our well-being—three of the richest human assets—for free. The resulting revolution in self-reliance and personal empowerment will transform medicine, business, and even our communities.

We can share with each other the health enhancement knowledge that we learn from our own experiences, the wisdom of our grandmothers, the secrets of ancient traditions, and the breakthroughs of new research. This kind of sharing has never required special training, mysterious abilities, expensive certification, or an academic diploma. The only necessary credential to participate in this revolution is the desire to improve oneself and help others. Our families and our communities will improve automatically as we sincerely improve ourselves.

Just as our elders shared remedies for healing their families in times past, we can share strategies for empowering each other in the present. The basic elements are really simple: self-respect, love for others, and the vision of a better world.

In over twenty years in the practice of medicine I have worked with thousands of people and their families. People have frequently asked, "Is there medicine in the acupuncture needles?" "No, these are not like needles you've experienced at the doctor's office before," I have replied. Then they typically ask, "Well, where is the medicine?" Usually I say, "Just relax and think it through." Later many have said, "I think I understand: the medicine is in me, isn't it?"

My experience of what average individuals can do to heal and empower themselves has excited and inspired me. Over and over real people like Patricia have proved to me that the most important medicine is not found in the doctor's office, the hospital, or the pharmacy. It is produced automatically within us. In those who are well this medicine within is in ample supply. In those who have lost their health, the healer within may be reactivated to produce this powerful self-healing medicine.

The self-healing and health enhancement methods in this book have evolved out of the programs for group study and support that we have conducted at the Health Action Clinic in Santa Barbara, California, for more than ten years. Gentle movement of the body, self-applied massage, regulation of the breath, and deep relaxation all have ancient roots. They have been refined and improved for thousands of years. Each is a powerful tool for activating the healer within. Along with these tools, a comprehensive program of personal health improvement, called PHASES (see page 246), also was developed at the Health Action Clinic.

Today the self-healing methods and the PHASES program, in conjunction with natural healing methods like acupuncture, massage, herbal medicine, and homeopathy, are being used in numerous hospitals, innovative clinics, and health maintenance programs throughout the world. Severely ill patients, health seekers, stressed executives, athletes, teachers, corporate employees, seniors, children, farmers—all types of people have learned to create their own personal plan for health enhancement, personal empowerment, and self-healing.

Yes, I am saying that the most profound medicine—a very real and powerful healing elixir—is produced within you! You can, using the simple methods you are about to learn, increase and improve the activity of this potent inner resource.

Take a moment to consider this deeply. If the most powerful healing resource is produced within ourselves and if it is possible purposefully to turn this elixir on, it then becomes reasonable to ask, "Who is the genuine healer, and where does the healer work?" Another good question is "How much does it cost to activate the genuine healer?"

A powerful medicine that is produced within us that does not require a doctor's prescription and has no cost—clearly, this idea is one of the "health wonders" of the world. It may honestly be the most extraordinary medical breakthrough in recent history, and it could completely transform medicine in the twenty-first century. Each person who learns to use the self-healing methods and then shares the secret of self-healing with others is a genuine hero.

By using the health enhancement and self-healing methods in this book, you automatically become a participant in a powerful, positive revolution that will have worldwide effects. Diseases that have been hard to cure, like cancer, heart disease, HIV, and diabetes, will become less devastating. Economies that have been terribly damaged by the cost of medicine will be rehabilitated. When the truths of self-reliance and self-healing are demonstrated person by person and community by community, a dynamic, widespread change will occur—a virtuous, wholesome, desirable, positive change.

This book opens the door to an exciting new realm. Use it as a first step in exploring traditional health enhancement and self-healing systems from around the world. Share your enthusiasm with others. No one person need be responsible for the possible worldwide effect of a self-healing revolution. Neither urgency, worry, nor anxiety is required. Simply take independent, calm, and deliberate action. You will be participating in a wave of change that will spontaneously multiply and radiate. Healing ourselves—and even healing the world—requires that we each be responsible only for the part of the world that lies within us.

What You'll Find in This Book

In this book you will find one set of powerful self-healing and health enhancement tools, eight life-transforming pearls of wisdom, and one radical future possibility.

The Tools

1 Gentle, purposeful movement of the body
2 Self-applied massage
3 Breathing practice
4 Deep relaxation, meditation, and prayer

The Pearls

1 The healer is within us.
2 We produce the most profound medicine ever developed in human history within our own bodies.
3 The self-healing and health enhancement methods turn these medicines on.
4 We can heal disease and enhance our vitality—for free.
5 We can transform the crisis in medicine into a rebirth of self-reliance.

6 The self-healing methods have hundreds of applications that can heal and empower our communities.

7 The practice of the self-healing methods can expand our spiritual practice.

8 Average people can teach each other to do self-healing.

The Possibility

1 Through our practice we contribute to a "healing field"; when we heal ourselves we help to heal the world.

How to Use This Book

Because every human being is unique, each of you will use this book differently. To begin the practice of awakening the healer and the medicines within immediately, go directly to part 2 on page 23 and explore the methods. To understand the pearls of wisdom, enjoy parts 1, 3, and 4 in any order and at your own pace. Those of you who are attracted to "the possibilities" will find them in part 5.

If you are so inspired by these ideas that you would like to participate in accelerating this revolution, the appendix offers ideas about how to share what you have learned with others. The appendix also provides some brief physiological explanations of how the healer within works and describes the use of herbs as a powerful supplement to the self-healing and health enhancement practices.

Remember, no matter what your level of interest, the starting place is always the same: embrace the practice. For those who are ill, for those who are well, and for those who are inspired to teach the self-healing and health enhancement methods to others, the essence is always the same: awaken the healer within, cultivate the medicine within, focus on the practice.

Who Will Benefit from This Book

"The Healer Within" dwells within all people. Those who are severely ill will benefit from this book as will those who are well but wish to be radiantly well and highly productive. Every disease or illness challenge can be improved by using these practices. They have helped to completely heal a wide array of disorders and they have helped to relieve the symptoms of many severe and even incurable diseases. A complete list of illnesses that have been improved through the practices in this book would run many pages. Whether you hope to cure disease, to relieve discomfort, or to create optimal health, try these simple tools; everyone benefits, you will be amazed.

Part 1

THE MEDICINE

It is the primary role of the physician, whether the African witch doctor or the modern doctor, to entertain the patient while secretly waiting for nature to heal the disease.

Albert Schweitzer,
physician, philosopher

o

How strange that we would produce the most profound medicine within our own bodies and then, somehow, forget to use it.

CHAPTER 1

Our Power of Self-Healing

*The marvelous pharmacy that was designed
by nature and placed into our being by the
universal architect produces most of the
medicines that we need.*

Norman Cousins,
editor, innovator, professor

YOUR BODY, IN COOPERATION WITH YOUR MIND AND
spirit, is marvelously blessed with miraculous self-healing abilities. The body is the temple of your life. Mind and spirit are the
dwellers within the temple. Mind and spirit maintain the temple.
Mind's intelligence and spirit's inspiration vitalize and quicken
the body. The three together—body, mind, and spirit—cooperate
to produce the most profound medicine ever known in the history of the human race, right within you.

Any injury or illness is spontaneously cured when these naturally occurring self-healing resources are operating optimally.
When you cut yourself, the wound heals automatically. When you
have a sprain or bruise, it heals automatically. When you have a
broken bone, the physician must set the bone correctly, but then
nature heals it spontaneously. The famous sixteenth-century
physician Ambroise Paré said, "I administered the treatment, but
nature provided the cure."

I had a personal revelation of this early in my own life. Through a series of sports accidents, one of my front teeth was broken off to half its length. While the planning for a cap for the tooth was in process, the tooth actually began to grow. Over six months this tooth called on inner resources to grow past its normal size until it was as long as the other, unbroken front tooth. Some unexplained interaction of forces and elements caused this unusual healing event to occur. Science cannot explain much of what causes what we call healing. The "original cause" of healing, health, life itself, and the whole universe is unexplained. In ancient China this "original cause" is known as "mystery."

An inside joke in medical circles reflects on the healing power of nature: "With a doctor's expert care you should be better in a week, but without access to the marvels of modern medicine your recovery will require at least seven days." With or without a physician, with or without medical intervention, the natural medicine that we produce—our healer within—is working to heal us and sustain our health.

A wondrous self-healing mechanism has been built into us by the architect of the universe from the beginning of human history. This remarkable gift belongs to every person from birth. Unfortunately, most people have not known about this gift; it has been a secret. You, however, have entered into the circle of individuals who will make this secret known. Freeing the potential of self-healing in your own life and sharing it with your family and community will have marvelous effects.

Once upon a time and for many thousands of years, humans did not have fire. Much later, when only a few had fire, it changed the course of human history dramatically. Keepers of the secret of how to produce fire had tremendous power. Then, in an extraordinary historical moment, fire became the property of the many, rather than the few. Now anyone powerful enough to ask for matches at the corner store can have fire for no cost.

You are involved in an equally extraordinary and historic moment. The period in human history around the year 2000 will be remembered as the phenomenal time when the secret of healing became the property of the many, rather than the few. Once, long ago, the secret of fire was known only to a few; later, people discovered how to mass-produce matches. Now, the keepers of the secret of healing have made an equally profound discovery: the essential resources for healing, which are naturally occurring within each individual, can be activated purposefully at no cost.

When our natural healing ability does not function automatically, something is terribly wrong. Our spontaneous self-healing resources have become damaged or disordered. Formerly, we lived in a world where the only solution to this problem was thought to require physicians, hospitals, medicines, and tremendous expense. Now we know that the best, easiest, and least expensive cure is to rehabilitate the automatic healing capacity through self-healing methods. The simple practices of focusing on the breath, applying self-massage, gently moving the body, and deeply relaxing bring the natural relationship among the body, mind, and spirit back into balance.

In mild cases like stress headache, occasional constipation, colds and flus, aches and pains, insomnia, and anxiety, these self-healing methods can completely replace the need for medication. When medicine is necessary, self-healing methods complement and support the treatment. Most medications or medical treatments do not actually restore or fully heal our natural ability to sustain a high level of well-being. In addition, the possible side effects of many medications are frightening. If we really think about it, most of what we have come to call health care does not authentically and actually improve health.

Medical pain relief and medical reduction of symptoms are not typically accomplished by enhancing health. The surgical removal of a section of the colon or heart bypass surgery, for example, may save a life and reduce pain. Such procedures even improve quality of life and comfort level. But it would be false to say that these surgeries genuinely restore the original health of the person.

The use of pain medication does not actually eliminate pain; it only eliminates the *sensation* of pain while, we hope, the spontaneous self-healing ability of the body is actually improving health and eliminating the *cause* of the pain. Only rarely will physicians disagree with this idea. Unfortunately, until recently it has also been rare for the medical community to focus on and encourage self-healing practices.

Spontaneous self-healing ability is not a dramatic new scientific discovery. Nor is it a "New Age" phenomenon. Many techniques and methods for self-healing are quite ancient. As we learned from Patricia's story, which demonstrated the healing power of the breath, relaxation, and faith, there are potent messages in the Judeo-Christian traditions regarding the healing resources that we have within ourselves. In China and India, as well as in Africa, ancient America, Australia, and Europe, rich traditions of self-care and self-healing have existed since long before written history. One of the first things I learned about in the study of traditional Chinese medicine was Qi (Chi), which is the name for the medicine within. The process of cultivating the medicine within is called Qigong (Chi Kung).

For decades, we in the modern Western world have believed that medical science would invent better medicines and healing procedures than those automatically born within us. Given that cancer, heart disease, stroke, and diabetes remain terrifying realities throughout our communities, we now know that the promise of medical science has been at least as much of a disappointment as it has been an inspiration. Exciting new scientific research and clinical experience show, however, that the most profound medicine is produced naturally within us through the collaboration of our own body, mind, and spirit.

Research of the U.S. Department of Health and Human Services, presented in the *Healthy People 2000* report, states that over 70 percent of all disease is preventable (DHHS, 1991). Recently, the *New England Journal of Medicine* reported that eight out of nine deaths occur from preventable causes (Fries, Koop, 1993). In 1996, on the eve of the one hundredth Olympic games, the office of the U.S. surgeon general confirmed that simple, mild exercise significantly decreases the risk of many serious diseases (DHHS, 1996). Sixty percent of adults were found to be insufficiently active, and 25 percent were found to be completely inactive. It was found that simply increasing physical activity a small amount has a powerful fitness-enhancing and disease-reducing effect.

It is obvious that self-care and prevention are preferable to medical intervention. Even our own folk traditions—the wisdom of our grandmothers—insists that "an ounce of prevention is better than a pound of cure" and "a stitch in time saves nine." When we take steps to sustain and enhance the mysterious "original cause" of vitality and health, medical intervention is necessary less often. Even in cases where health has been lost and where pain and disease have set in, self-care can lead to dramatic recovery.

Think of it: if 70 percent of each medical dollar were saved through self-reliance and prevention, the U.S. annual medical bill of nearly one trillion dollars would be cut to three hundred billion dollars. Perhaps 20 percent would become the cost of prevention, so the savings would amount to five hundred billion dollars. That kind of savings would be a huge step toward a more creative and reasonable economy, which could support other needs in education, repair of bridges and roads, research, and the renewal of our communities. Just imagine having access to five hundred billion dollars.

Here is a perfect place to take a deep, relaxed breath.

If it was extremely difficult or impossible to sustain health through the personal practice of self-care and self-healing, then perhaps we would have to live with these immense medical costs. It turns out, however, that the process of turning on the natural medicine within ourselves is not a difficult one. In fact, it is easy, user friendly, and free.

The naturally occurring self-healing ability of your own body, mind, and spirit is the world's greatest healer. This means that you—not someone else, but you—can reduce your risk of disease. If you have lost your health and have become challenged by a disease or illness, this means that you can literally heal yourself. Or you can work as a partner with your physician to speed your recovery.

This also means that your best health insurance is to be sure that all of the self-healing mechanisms within you are operating optimally. This does not suggest that our physicians will no longer be needed. Nor does it suggest that the medical advances of the last one hundred years are any less remarkable. But it does mean that our physicians' time could be used more effectively in dealing with the 30 percent of health problems that are not preventable. And when it is necessary to have expert medical care, we can work as partners with our physicians and therapists by purposefully stimulating our own precious gift of self-healing.

The Essence of Self-Healing

The physician who teaches people to sustain their health is the superior physician. The physician who waits to treat people until after their health is lost is considered to be inferior. This is like waiting until one's family is starving to begin to plant seeds in the garden.
Yellow Emperor's Classic on Internal Medicine, 500 B.C.E.

Three areas, all based on personal choice and personal action, maximize the activity of our naturally occurring self-healing capability. The first is our choice of attitudes and mental influences. When we choose to think, believe, and act from a position of power, refusing to be a victim of circumstances, the healer within is automatically strengthened. When we refuse to live under the influence of worry and doubt, the internal medicine is enriched.

The second area of choice is lifestyle: nutrition, exercise, rest, relationships, finances, work, spiritual practice, play, water intake, avoidance of alcohol and cigarettes, and so on. From moment to moment, each of us personally elects whether to enhance or sabotage the healer within through our behaviors and personal choices. In my practice of acupuncture and Chinese medicine I have found that the people who dislike their work, don't take time to play, or have poor self-esteem and communication skills are typically the most difficult patients to treat successfully. In such cases the acupuncture often activates the healer within, but then the person's life situation tends to neutralize the self-healing capacity.

Around 1983 at the Health Action Clinic in Santa Barbara, we began to redesign our health care delivery and the flow of our clinical activities. This led to the development of a program that focuses in a holistic way on attitudes and lifestyle. This program, now called PHASES, assists people in making better choices in their attitudes and lifestyles and in reaching for greater health, mastery of stress, and improved personal effectiveness. It is complementary to the natural healing modalities of acupuncture, massage, and herbal medicine. It rests on the idea that people improve in "phases," rather than all at once.

We have found that patients, corporate employees, teachers, bankers, and athletes are always genuinely excited about improving their health and performance. Healthy people have more fun and have the creative energy to respond to new opportunities. Healthy people have energy left after work so that they can balance their life with play. High-performance people have the vitality and endurance for dynamic living. They often make more money. Who would turn down the chance to feel better, be healthier, or have more energy?

The third area of choice is personal self-care—the practice of self-healing and health enhancement methods. This area of choice for improving, sustaining, and ensuring the function of the healer within is the primary subject of this book. The self-applied health enhancement methods (SAHEM) and the attitude and lifestyle program (PHASES) are like brother and sister. They complement and enhance each other. The interaction of these three choice areas—attitudes, lifestyle, and self-care—is becoming and will remain the foundation of health care and healing deep into the twenty-first century.

When these aspects of personal choice keep health and healing active in a person's life, he or she does not generally need to go to a clinic or hospital. When the healer within is strong and efficient, well-being is intact. Empowered by knowledge and inspiration to take action, each individual becomes the principal source of health, healing, and stress mastery in his or her own life.

The status of attitude, lifestyle, and self-care is noticeable in people's lives. For example, it is fairly obvious when an individual is under the influence of self-doubt, poor nutrition, and no health enhancement practice. It is equally obvious when an individual is influenced by enthusiasm, purposeful work, and the regular practice of health enhancement methods. The first person is typically exhausted and frustrated, the other is radiant and energetic. One is a victim, the other is a leader and a role model. One is part of the problem, the other is part of the solution.

To accelerate our naturally occurring healing capability is actually quite easy. Once we replace the idea that health improvement comes from external sources with the knowledge that healing can come from the healer within, the practice of self-applied health enhancement methods is simply logical.

The Four Essential Methods

In addition to following basic guidelines in the areas of attitude and lifestyle, each individual can learn and practice four simple self-applied health enhancement methods that activate the natural medicines that we produce within. These are ancient practices. After many centuries of correction and improvement, they have become highly refined tools.

1 Gentle movement of the body
2 Self-applied massage
3 Breath practice
4 Deep relaxation or meditation

These techniques are easy to learn, are easy to apply, require no special knowledge or training, and can be practiced daily by all people (sick or well) with little impact on their time or energy. In fact, they will actually produce both time and energy. The methods create time because they reduce or eliminate fatigue and forgetfulness. They generate energy because they enhance and regenerate the functioning of the organs and glands, and this produces the physiological energy needed for activity and endurance.

The time spent applying these methods will be returned, even multiplied, by your growing ability to generate abundant personal vitality, balance, and well-being. You will waste less time and need less sleep. For every fifteen minutes of health enhancement practice, done faithfully for a period of days, fifteen minutes less sleep will be required, fifteen minutes less time looking for lost keys will be needed, fifteen minutes less insomnia or depression will be experienced, fifteen minutes less pain relief from over-the-counter pain medications will be necessary, fifteen minutes less time will be spent in the waiting room of the doctor's office or clinic.

Recently, I received a phone call from a woman who had attended a training in these self-healing methods in Chicago. At the workshop she complained that she didn't think she had the time to do the practices every day. She didn't discuss the details of her medical problems, but her doctor was evidently trying different medications, probably to regulate blood pressure or manage anxiety.

During our brief telephone conversation she was very excited: "I figured out where to get the time to do the practices. I took you at your word and have practiced the methods every day for twenty to forty-five minutes. It takes almost half a day to keep a doctor's appointment, about four hours—getting to her office, finding parking, waiting for my appointment (she often runs late), having a brief visit with no time for questions, going to the pharmacy, and then driving home.

"Now that I am doing the self-healing methods, I'm feeling better. The doctor needs to see me less. She has started cutting back on my medicine. In a month's time I used to spend, I think, about fifteen hours going to the doctor, sitting in traffic, going to the drugstore, and taking pills. That's just about how much time I am now spending doing the self-healing methods. I certainly prefer doing the practices at home or at the park near my house to all that running around."

In recent years thousands of people have learned the simple methods you are about to learn. Many have experienced dramatic health improvement, sometimes very quickly. There are some cases where people have felt better in the first ten to fifteen minutes. With a week or so of repetition of the methods, most people are able to feel a definite shift in their body within just a few minutes of beginning their daily practice. In many cases individuals have experienced "being better" in as little as ten to fifteen days. Everyone who has been vigilant with these simple practices has experienced some level of health improvement. The key word here is *vigilant.*

Real People's Stories

The multitudes of cases that I have observed personally and clinically over twenty years of practice as a physician are a powerful testimony to the possibilities of self-initiated healing. Please refer to page 187, where the healing potential of testimonial is explained. And scientific research in the United States as well as in

China, Europe, and Japan has now confirmed that relaxation, deep breathing, gentle movement, and self-massage are excellent health improvement tools. (Please refer to the bibliography and suggested reading section for these references in the literature.)

Until you actually begin to meet people face to face who have had positive experiences with self-healing, it will help to meet some people here who have used these methods. Allow me to tell you just a few stories to help inspire you until you have begun to practice the methods yourself. Several of these are stories of people who have attended a Wednesday practice session that met weekly for a number of years.

In just one practice session, Sara, a nurse from Ventura, California, eliminated uncomfortable gastric acid reflux (burning acid in the throat) that had been constant since the birth of her last baby over twenty years before. She had tried numerous medical solutions, including a long list of medicines. She commented that self-massage of the abdominal area (see "Massaging the Abdomen," page 72), following her practice of the self-healing methods in general, was the key ingredient.

At the annual conference of the National Wellness Institute at the University of Wisconsin, I presented a brief workshop on self-applied massage. After the initial session I was reading through the evaluations and was particularly gratified to find this one: "This simple class on self-massage relieved my eye pain! I've had two surgeries and the MDs don't 'see' the reason for the pain, which is severe and continuous. After this brief class my pain is significantly reduced."

A young man with AIDS gave a wonderful testimonial at a recent International Conference on HIV/AIDS and Chinese Medicine at Columbia University. He said that two of his main problems were an inability to quit smoking and difficulty with insomnia. On the first day of the conference he was in a one-hour class on some of the simple Chinese methods of self-applied health enhancement. He returned on the second day quite excited. He reported that during the class he'd had a strong impression that he should incorporate the practices into his daily routine. That night he had done just ten minutes of the practices. The cigarette that he'd had before bed, he said, tasted awful and made him gag: "I believe the self-care practices must awaken some natural body wisdom, because I have smoked for years and never had that reaction." He also reported that his sleep improved dramatically. Instead of lying awake for an hour or more and then continuing to wake up throughout the night, which was his usual experience, he fell right to sleep and "slept like a baby the whole night through."

An innovative occupational therapist from Arizona incorporated some of the methods with difficult emphysema clients and found that a number of them experienced significant improvement immediately. The rehabilitation hospital where she worked decided to train all of the occupational and physical therapy staff in using and teaching the self-applied health enhancement methods. Occupational therapists are particularly well suited to bringing these methods into the health care system, since health insurance companies can be billed for the strategies that they use to help patients improve their daily living capabilities.

Maria, a psychotherapist from San Diego, found the training in the health enhancement and self-healing methods so inspiring that she implemented some of the practices in both her areas of professional expertise. At the UCLA Asthma Control and Treatment Center, a combination of breathing techniques, relaxation practices, and gentle body movements helped her adolescent asthma patients break through to new levels of personal control and comfort.

Her favorite testimonial came from her experience with one of her clients in another program at an agency for developmentally retarded individuals. He had a terrible and uncontrollable urge to hit others. He was documented by the case manager as having up to one hundred episodes a month of hitting, occasionally vigorously. Maria taught this young man a set of specific steps to use when he experienced the urge to hit. The steps included deepening the breath, relaxing purposefully, and making specific gentle movements of the hands and arms that were coordinated with his breathing. In a short time he began to gain control of his hitting behavior.

At first, others were terrified because the breathing method and hand motions that he was using sounded and looked like he was revving up to attack. However, he was actually in the process of redirecting his internal impulses, and his use of the self-healing techniques was eventually a huge success, offering relief to every-one in the program. In just the first eight weeks of practice, he brought the number of hitting episodes down to fewer than fif-teen a month, and over time he was able to curtail the hitting be-havior almost completely.

Adele, who had attended many of the weekly practice sessions in Santa Barbara, was a volunteer doing blood pressure screening at a community recreation center. She reported one week that she had decided to see if any of the people she worked with could lower their blood pressure using the health enhancement meth-ods. One gentleman whose pressure was significantly elevated agreed to rub his ears (page 65) for a few minutes and take a num-ber of deep relaxed breaths. She was surprised to find that in just that brief period his pressure came down twenty-five points.

A physicist named Bob who "loves to play with ideas" told his story in 1995 to an audience of physicians during my presentation at the First International Conference on Alternative and Comple-mentary Medicine in Washington, D.C. He had a difficult heart problem and a history of several emergency hospitalizations. His physicians had urged him to lose weight. Several special diets had not helped him, but when he began to do the breathing practices more frequently, he began to lose weight. As a scientist he was very meticulous about the process and insists that the only change in his daily lifestyle and activities during this period was his focus on the breathing practices. He became so enthusiastic that he began to devise a system for remembering to breathe deeply throughout the day (see "The Remembering Breath," page 89). He has documented 107 daily activities that he can do that help him remember to deepen his breath. His doctor has agreed that he has eliminated the need for any medication, and Bob still calls me occasionally to report new breakthroughs in his practice of self-healing.

In some cases, vigilance has been a primary key to success. After several years of simple daily practice, numerous people have said, "I would have been dead or incapacitated a long time ago, but instead I am alive and feeling better than I have felt in years." Elizabeth's is one such story.

At eighty years old, Elizabeth says that before beginning to use the self-applied health enhancement methods she could not sit up to get out of bed. Each day she would literally crawl from the bed to the bathroom. She had significant osteoarthritis and numerous heart complications following triple bypass heart surgery. Following the death of her husband, Roy, everything got worse and she fell into a severe depression.

She found acupuncture and massage to be helpful but declares that she was mostly inspired by the idea that she could regain her health through self-care. She first discovered the self-healing methods at a class that was cosponsored by Valley Community Hospital and the Santa Barbara community adult education program. She has been loyal to the weekly practice sessions for several years, but the most powerful key to her recovery has been her vigilant daily practice at home.

As Elizabeth likes to say, "I taught young children for many years and delighted in their constant activity. Being joyful and active was the center of my life. Following the death of my husband and that intense surgery I was so low and uncomfortable and lifeless that I am surprised I survived. My doctors didn't know what to do with me; they had already done what they know to do. Through natural healing, especially the self-healing practices, I have literally been reborn.

"I start doing the self-healing methods before I get out of bed. One of the most important for me is the special back exercise that I do lying down [Right and Left Bending of the Spine, page 40]; it really changed the pain in my ribs. I try to do the Remembering Breath [page 89] as often as possible throughout the day; I walk by the sea; I do some of the Front and Back Bending of the Spine [page 44] in my backyard while the sunset lights up the mountains. My favorite is the Flowing Motion [page 37]; I do a few of them several times throughout the day. I'm healthier than I've been in years and still improving. I'm even buying a new house in Utah and going on a trip to Alaska. What a marvel: I'm still alive long after I thought I would have passed away."

Formula for Making Miracles

Our friends and neighbors are learning to complement their medical treatment with self-healing methods. They are learning to increase their vitality and master the stress in their lives.

Knowledge of the healer within is spreading. It is no longer a secret. It is moving from the few to the many.

There is a brief and simple formula for self-healing and health enhancement: *Awaken the medicine within, restore the natural self-healing capacity of body, mind, and spirit.* One of the most effective ways to activate this formula is the regular practice of the four essential self-care methods.

CHAPTER 2

Placebos, Remissions, and Miracles

There must be some primal force,
but it is impossible to find.
I believe it exists, but cannot see it.
I see its results,
I can even feel it,
But it has no form.

Chang Tsu, philosopher, poet,
fourth century B.C.E.

THE PLACEBO EFFECT, SPONTANEOUS REMISSIONS, AND miracles provide rich food for thought regarding the healer within and the self-healing resources upon which we can draw. In each of these areas, healing occurs where no medical intervention has been utilized or where medical intervention has failed. By exploring the research on placebos, remissions, and miracles we confirm the power of our self-healing potential. We verify that a dynamic healing resource is produced spontaneously within the individual. We can supercharge our self-healing practice by understanding that spontaneous healing is not merely a hope or possibility. Healing without medicines or medical procedures is a documented reality.

The Placebo

The placebo is the doctor that resides within.

Norman Cousins

In 1983 I was invited to give a lecture on the medicine within to the Annual Medical Symposium in Phoenix, Arizona. In preparing for that presentation, I looked again at the scientific literature on the placebo, which I believe is one of the strongest bodies of knowledge confirming our self-healing capacity.

The concept of placebo has been through several dramatic phases just in recent history. Placebo means literally, in Latin, "to please." In the 1800s and early 1900s the term *placebo* described substances that appeared to be medicines but had no clinical action. Physicians would frequently administer a placebo, usually a sugar pill, when the patient's natural healing process was progressing positively, and nature just needed a little more time to resolve the disorder. Such remedies were also used to please patients who insisted on receiving medicine when it was not necessary.

Between 1920 and the present, the use of placebo remedies fell from favor. The word was then used in the phrase "placebo effect" to describe a process in clinical research. In medical research the response of two groups is compared. One group receives the medicine or surgical procedure that is being studied. The second, the control group, receives an inert substance that appears to be the medicine or a surgical procedure but actually has no clinical effect. If the group that receives the actual medicine or procedure has results that are significantly better than those of the control group, then it is assumed that it is clinically effective. A significant percentage of those who do not receive the actual drug or procedure typically experience improvement as well. The conventional view has been that 30 to 35 percent of any group would experience some improvement (Beecher, 1955). This is called the placebo effect. Patients who responded positively to inert substances or positive suggestion were termed "placebo reactors." During this period of history when self-healing was considered impossible, the placebo effect was a nuisance to scientists.

In a unique review of data from several older studies on innovative treatments for asthma, ulcers, and herpes simplex, researchers from Scripps's Clinic and Research Foundation discovered that 40 percent of patients reported "excellent" results, 30 percent reported "good" results, and only another 30 percent reported "poor" results—in other words, combining the "excellent" and "good" reports, there was a 70 percent effective rate (Roberts, 1995). This is generally considered to be solid confirmation that a medicine is clinically effective. Interestingly, however, these therapies were later found to be useless. This means that 70 percent of the patients had actually exhibited the power of the placebo. Their "excellent" and "good" healing results were due completely to the medicine within.

Dr. Bernie Siegel, author of *Love, Medicine, and Miracles* and *Peace, Love, and Healing,* was asked to comment on the placebo during his term as president of the American Holistic Medical Association. "The placebo effect," he said, "can change the body chemistry, change the internal hormones. It shows that mind and body are a single unit. If you read a chemotherapy protocol with all of its side effects to a patient, and then inject him with saline [no medicine, just a weak salt solution], the patient's hair falls out!!"

One hundred years ago doctors used placebos intentionally to mobilize the healer within. Then, more recently, using the placebo became a sign of quackery. It was a nuisance that complicated experimental data. Now, the placebo is finally gaining attention as proof that the healer within is authentic. The placebo is helping to redefine medicine and healing in terms that declare the power of self-healing resources.

Spontaneous Remission

The mechanisms of vis medicatrix naturae—*the healing power of nature—are so effective that most diseases are self-terminating.*
                              Rene Dubos, bacteriologist, philosopher

"Spontaneous remission" is the phrase typically used in the medical literature to describe cases in which a disease is cured or resolved but no one understands how. In the decades to come, the mechanism for spontaneous remission will be vigorously explored and will probably be better understood. For now it is not so important how it happens; it is just enlightening that it does happen.

When doctors acknowledge that a cure has occurred and then acknowledge that they don't know how, it is possible that internal healing resources have been spontaneously activated to cause the cure. In the 1980s, the Institute of Noetic Sciences decided to explore the remission concept as a possible strategy to confirm the human capacity for self-healing. Brendan O'Regan, then the vice president of research, began a systematic exploration of the medical literature for references to remission. To everyone's amazement he found an immense number of references: three thousand articles from over 860 medical journals in twenty languages. Some of the articles discussed hundreds of cases, so the overall number of cases actually reported in the literature turned out to be in the many thousands.

"We have many cases of remission (one-fifth of all cases)," O'Regan reported, "with no medical intervention at all. These are the purest ones, the ones that give us the strongest evidence that there is an extraordinary self-repair system lying dormant within us" (O'Regan, 1995). This historic analysis of the "remission" literature from the Institute of Noetic Sciences is a powerful confirmation of the healer within.

As a part of their research, the Noetic Sciences team actually tracked down a few of the people from the remission literature who were still living. Their insight offers powerful teachings for our work with the self-healing methods. One of the cancer cases felt it was critical to "keep my state of mind intact, no matter what." Another case, when asked what he attributed his cancer remission to, stated, "I really think it is our life, the way we experience our life." This person reported the value of daily meditation, spousal support, massage, acupuncture, Yoga, vegetarian diet, and colon cleansing.

These stories are usually called testimonials; like the placebo, testimonials have not been in favor until very recently. They were historically seen as unprovable. However, these are the stories of people documented in the scientific literature to have experienced the spontaneous remission of a dangerous disorder. The "stories" of people in remission prove, perhaps even as powerfully as science, that self-healing is an undeniable and obtainable promise.

Miracles

There are two ways to live your life. One is as though there are no miracles. The other is as though everything is a miracle.

Albert Einstein

The capacity to produce a healing resource, an elixir, within ourselves is a kind of miracle. To some, a miracle is a natural occurrence that we do not yet have the knowledge to understand. George Santayana, a modern philosopher, noted, "Miracles are fortunate accidents, the natural causes of which are too complicated to be readily understood." Certainly, the ability to fly would have been considered a miracle in previous eras; now air travel is a common occurrence that is readily understood. By the early twenty-first century, it is likely that the miracle of self-healing will be better understood as well.

There is a second view of miracles that points to the supernatural and the divine. Miraculous outcomes credited to God's love and to angelic presences are very common throughout history. In a fascinating study of miracles, Carolyn Miller, Ph.D., has looked into hundreds of unexplainable situations. In her book, *Creating Miracles: Understanding the Experience of Divine Intervention,* she concludes that miracles are frequently supernatural events. She was able to condense, out of numerous real cases, a formula for eligibility for a miracle. She calls it "miracle mindedness": "Inner peace leads to miracles, the decision to shift into a loving, peaceful, accepting mental state is a necessary precondition for miracles, miracles do not produce faith, faith produces miracles." In the Book of Luke in the Christian Bible, Jesus says, "Don't be afraid, just believe and she will be healed." The formula asks that we be at peace. This, in some way, creates the possibility for a miracle.

In our quest to understand self-healing and the empowering resources that we spontaneously produce within, we do not need to know exactly how miracles work. It is enough to know that they actually occur. The shrine of the Virgin Mary at Lourdes in France marks the place where an apparition of the Holy Virgin appeared in 1858. Since then, over six thousand claims of miraculous healing have occurred. It is easy enough for miraculous claims to be made, but how do you prove a miracle?

In 1947 an official commission was formed to determine whether actual miracles were occurring. The twenty-five-member International Medical Commission is made up of medical professionals from a broad array of medical specialties from nine countries. They follow a strict eighteen-point protocol. Among other points, a correct diagnosis must have been made, the disease must be serious, no sign of psychosomatic influence can be present, medical treatment must have failed completely, the cure must be fully confirmed, and the time since the cure must be significant.

With this rigorous set of guidelines in place, sixty-four "certified miracles" have been documented. The twenty-five physician members of the International Medical Commission have agreed that there is no way that these cases could have achieved a cure without some unknown influence that operated in a way contrary to the observations and expectations of medical knowledge. The cures include the disappearance of tumors, blindness, paralysis, and even the regrowth of bone in a case where the hip joint had deteriorated so severely that the leg and pelvis had become separated.

Miraculous healings may be natural events that we cannot yet understand. Or miracles may be direct interventions by supernatural forces, angels, or God. In either case the healing occurs by the mysterious mobilization of natural resources within the person.

We are at an extraordinary turning point in human development. Science has begun honestly to explore mysterious concepts that until recently were considered unscientific. Shining the light of science on the placebo, spontaneous remission, and miracles has demonstrated that the mysterious can be verified even if it is not understood. It is exciting to know that the placebo has taken on a positive definition, that one-fifth of the cases in three thousand medical articles on remission are "pure," and that a twenty-five-member international team using an eighteen-point criterion has found sixty-four "certified miracles" at Lourdes.

Placebo, remission, and miracles are areas of radical breakthrough. They change the rules. They confirm the presence of the healer within. They suggest that our practice of self-healing methods can mobilize the internal capacity for self-repair. And they point to the value of the body, mind, and spirit interaction.

Part 2

THE TOOLS AND METHODS

Give people loaves of bread, and you have fed them for a day.

Teach people to plant seeds, harvest grain, and bake bread, and you have fed them for a lifetime.

Ancient proverb

O

The self-applied health enhancement methods are simple self-healing tools with powerful roots in ancient healing traditions as well as in modern science. They will create a dramatic revolution in the history of health care and medicine. They cost nothing, cause no negative side effects, and may be used any time and anywhere by anyone.

CHAPTER 3

Your Personal Practice

Practice is the supreme teacher.

Publilius Syrus,
Greek philosopher, first century

DOZENS OF SPONTANEOUS SELF-HEALING MECHANISMS,
such as the blood's delivery of oxygen and nutrition to the cells,
the lymph's removal of waste products from the tissues, and the
brain's secretion of chemicals that accelerate immune and other
functions, are all programmed to sustain or restore our health
and vitality automatically. But they must be operating fully and
freely. The self-applied health enhancement methods enrich and
accelerate the capacity of the blood, lymph, immune system, neurochemistry, and other self-healing mechanisms to do their jobs.
(The appendix describes in more detail how this occurs.)

The raw materials for your personal health enhancement and
self-healing practice have roots in many different traditions. The
methods you will be learning come from ancient self-healing systems, philosophies of natural healing, folk practices with European
roots, Asian medical traditions, the wisdom of our grandmothers,
recent scientific breakthroughs, and my own experiences as a
physician. Eventually, no matter what sources you draw on, your
practice will be modified by your own experience.

Each of the "how to" chapters that follow will empower you to
learn, practice, and share the self-healing and health enhancement

methods. These chapters form a remarkable tool kit with multiple applications. The methods can be healing tools, health maintenance tools, stress mastery tools, productivity tools, and even survival tools. You choose. Throughout the book you will find examples of how these methods are used in hospitals, schools, churches, and corporations. Notice that the same simple methods are adaptable to a great variety of settings. In part 3 you will learn how to draw from these resources to assemble brief or extended practice sessions. There are literally hundreds of variations and modifications to ease and enhance the use of these tools.

There is just one critical detail: you must actually remember to do the practices. We remember to tune into our favorite TV shows and seek our favorite desserts. We repeat behaviors like cleaning our teeth and bathing our bodies. The human being has the built-in capability to create and sustain certain habits. Over time it will become easy to remember these practices. They will become a new habit for you. The key is to allow time, assign time, or take time in your day for self-healing action: ten to fifteen minutes at a regular time each day, perhaps before breakfast, at lunch, or even during commercials on TV. It can be that simple. Add a few moments of conscious practice—breathing and deep relaxation—just before sleep and for a moment when you awaken in the morning.

Once you begin, your doubts will fade away. After just a little daily practice you will begin to feel the transformation in your life. Your practice of these methods will provide its own confirming feedback.

Guidelines for Your Practice

Several guidelines will help make these life-enhancing tools most effective. They will help to keep both your interest and fun levels high, without taking up much of your time:

○ Do some of these practices every day. Put them at the core of your life and build the rest of your daily activities around them. Consider them as important in your day as you do rest, bathing, and dental hygiene. This will guarantee you the best results.

○ Keep your practice simple and fun. Start with a few of the methods and add as you wish. If you push to do too much, these

simple but powerful activities could become stressors for you
and thus become more of a problem than a solution. So keep
things simple and light as you begin.

o Make up your own system, adapting the order, number, and pace
of the methods to accommodate your personal situation. Be the
inventor of your practice. Nothing is new under the sun; all of
this was created and arranged by someone at sometime in history. Now it is your turn to invent it to fit yourself.

o Seek guidance and support, but avoid highly regimented systems
and methods whose teachers infer that their approach is the
"only" way. You are the greatest expert in your life. Allow your
practice to help you become your own best teacher. The practice
itself is the supreme teacher.

o Find the right attire for your practice. You want to be neither hot
nor cool. Seek balance and comfort.

o Find the perfect spot for your practice. Generally people prefer
an outdoor spot—in the park, in the yard, or on the patio—but a
spot in your bedroom or den may be best for you. Only you
know where to be. Set yourself up to succeed. If going outside
seems a strain, then know that your perfect spot is inside.

o Experiment with different times throughout the day for your primary practice. Most people find it easier to do it first thing, before the busyness of the day takes over. This way you won't end
up saying, "I'll do my self-healing practice as soon as I have finished this or that." If this or that does not get done, then you will
never practice. This is why the Chinese go into the parks at 5:30
or 6:00 A.M. Thirty minutes early in the day and then little bits of
practice integrated here and there can equal an hour of practice.
It's OK to do less; you could start with just ten or fifteen minutes
for health maintenance. More is better for improving health or
healing an illness. *If you are ill, please start slowly.*

o Do not leave the comfort zone. Increase the intensity of your
practice only when it feels easy to do so. Build or regenerate
yourself slowly. Success in these practices is not gained by ag-
gressive or compulsive practice. The only useful breakthrough is
when you grasp this vision: "I can transform myself." Victory occurs as you gently accelerate the naturally occurring self-healing
capability that you were born with. Don't go so far or so fast that
you overdo it and create a reason for discontinuing the practice.

○ Look for opportunities to practice with others. Notice that there is a growing movement for the practice of self-healing methods throughout the country and the world. People always comment that practicing in a group increases the effectiveness of the methods. In China it is believed that people practicing in groups create a "field" of healing energy that participants can draw on. Practice with others and see what you notice.

○ Focus on relaxing. The foundation of all self-healing, health enhancement, stress mastery, and personal empowerment is deep relaxation. In every aspect of your practice and in everything you do, relax.

Applications and Benefits

Following each of the methods is a section that makes suggestions for its application and describes its benefits. The application strategies are guidelines, not rules. They are intended to assist and guide you without inhibiting your creativity and freedom. Use the application suggestions to help you find your own inner sense of what works for you, and then adapt the suggestions according to your insight. Within each person there is a wisdom. You know your needs, likes, and limitations. No one can know these better than you do. Find your inner sense; follow its wisdom.

Application Suggestions

The application suggestions are divided into the following categories:

○ Health maintenance: This is the suggested practice level for sustaining health when you are a relatively healthy person.

○ Health improvement: This is the suggested practice level when you are only mildly unwell or if you are ill with a chronic or degenerative disorder.

○ Disease intervention: When you are severely unwell or challenged with serious disease, start *slowly* and build up to higher levels of practice. More practice can be better—but only when you have built a foundation of strength from beginning gently.

o Getting started: If you are well and strong, you may start with a vigorous daily practice. Suggestions for "getting started" are for those who are beginning these practices from a point of weakness, sickness, or diminished health.

Benefits

The section on benefits will generally contain a statement about physiological effects that are triggered by the practice. Because some practices produce unique benefits and others do not, this section will appear only when *unique* benefits can be expected. Thus, each of the movement practices creates a different benefit and has a separate "Benefits" section. All of the relaxation practices create similar benefits, however, and so only one section is necessary to accompany a number of relaxation practices.

The benefits are stated in simple terms, and in most cases they will actually be more extensive than those described. There are some possible benefits that science does not yet understand. If the Asian cultures are correct about the self-healing energy called Qi (Chi) and Prana—the energy that we might call the "life force"—then a whole array of benefits that we cannot yet explain scientifically are being gained through the self-applied health enhancement methods.

The Sensation of the Healer Within

With experience you may begin to actually feel the activity of your internal resources healing or energizing you. People experience the healer within in a variety of ways: "tingling," "warmth," "flowing," "humming," "fluffy," "light." Some people call the sensation of the inner medicine "restful," "calm," or "tranquil."

Interestingly, many people do not experience these sensations. Having such sensations is not particularly important. When you take a deep breath, it pumps the lymphatic aspect of the elimination system, whether you feel it or not. When you relax deeply, it shifts the mix of chemicals in the brain and endocrine glands, whether you feel it or not.

The Chinese say that this sensation is the Qi circulating in the body's energy channels. This dynamic life energy is always present.

A fish is not always aware of the water; we are not always aware of the air or the Qi. However, if you quiet the mind and deeply relax it is possible to sense the healing resources within.

Four Methods, One Integrated Practice

The four preliminary methods of health enhancement and self-healing can be learned and practiced as individual techniques, or they can be combined. When gentle body movements, self-massage, breath practice, and deep relaxation are integrated into a single practice, they become even more powerful. The Chinese and the Asian Indians have integrated and refined these methods for thousands of years. This integration also saves time, which is so precious to most people in Western culture.

In China the integration of these methods is called Qigong (Chi Kung), meaning "vitality enhancement practice." In India it is called Yoga. Both of these Asian traditions of self-healing have been called "internal exercises," "moving meditation," or "meditation in motion." In China, millions of people practice these methods daily. Children in schools, workers in factories, elders in the parks, and patients in hospitals all faithfully implement the self-applied health enhancement methods every day. Taiji (Tai Chi), which is familiar to many Americans and Europeans, is one kind of Qigong.

It is almost automatic that relaxation accompanies a deep breath. However, by adding the *intention* to relax to the breathing the result is even greater. Adding gentle movement does not require much additional concentration or effort, especially when the movements are simple and mild. It is also relatively easy to add deep breathing and relaxation to self-applied massage.

When deep breathing and relaxation are added to movement or massage, a special self-healing and health-generating state is created. It is this special state that so dramatically differentiates these methods from the more vigorous fitness methods typical in the Western world.

Integrated practice also points to the interaction of body, mind, emotions, and spirit. The focus on deep and intentful relaxation creates a shift in the body chemistry. The internal quiet and tranquillity allow for busyness to diminish and natural spirituality to arise. In some forms of self-healing practice Qigong or Yoga is used to help release emotional stress by linking body movement with voice sounds as in Sigh of Relief (page 92). The integration of movement, breath, and voice helps to integrate and balance the body, mind, and emotions.

Weaving the Practices into Your Day

Learning the four preliminary health enhancement methods is a powerful step toward greater health and productivity. They are most effective when they are woven into our daily lives. There are hundreds of opportunities throughout the day to integrate some combination of health enhancement methods into your activities. Here are some examples:

○ You are sitting at a stoplight. Take a deep breath.
○ You are just about to fall asleep or you have just awakened. Breathe deeply, and allow your whole body to become completely relaxed; place your hands together over your navel.
○ You are in the shower washing your hair. As you apply shampoo or conditioner, massage your scalp vigorously. Rub your ears, relax, take several deep breaths.
○ You are standing in line at the bank. Use the Flowing Motion (page 37), but modify it by minimizing the arm movement so that it is not obvious to others. Rise slowly up on your toes, breathe deeply, relax. Lift your fingers just slightly. Do it several times. You will find that nobody really notices or seems to care.
○ You are watching television. During each commercial break, alternate rubbing your hands, feet, and ears (page 61). Breathe deeply, relax. This is an easy way to affect your whole body without changing your schedule.
○ You are watering the garden. Put the hose near the first tomato plant or fruit tree, and do several repetitions of one of the methods in the "Gentle Movement" chapter (chapter 4). Combine them with deep breaths and the intention to relax deeply. Move the hose to the next plant. Do a few more repetitions.
○ You are hoeing the garden. Coordinate the movements of the hoe with the breath. Be conscious of your posture.
○ You are vacuuming the house. Relax your shoulders, breathe deeply, and coordinate your movements with your breathing.

○ You are working at the office. Every twenty minutes or so, take three deep breaths and gently adjust your posture. Notice that you automatically relax on the exhalation. Replace stressful thoughts with encouraging inner dialogue.

○ You are on the phone (possibly on hold). Give your free ear or shoulder some massage. Or take a few deep breaths.

○ You work as a checker in a grocery store. Make a deal with yourself that on greeting each new customer you will take a deep breath. Make a second deal: you will minimize your risk for carpal tunnel syndrome by faithfully doing the health enhancement practices every day.

○ You are on your daily walk. Add the In, Out Breathing (page 93). Literally millions of people use these methods every day in China.

These suggestions are just a small sample; there are many ways to bring these self-healing methods into your life. As you will see in part 3, the best strategy is to set aside specific times in your day. As little as ten to fifteen minutes of daily practice can have immense and immediate benefits. Even ten seconds here and there will create a positive change, awakening the healer within (see Momentary Methods, page 122). Weaving the methods into your daily activities multiplies and enhances the effectiveness of your practice.

CHAPTER 4

Method 1
Gentle Movement

Worms will not eat living wood where the vital sap is flowing; rust will not hinder the opening of a gate when the hinges are used each day.
Movement gives health and life. Stagnation brings disease and death.

Ancient proverb in traditional
Chinese medicine

NEAR THE END OF THE TWENTIETH CENTURY WESTERN science finally "discovered" something that has been common knowledge in the "less developed" cultures for thousands of years: consistent, mild fitness practice is a powerful healing and health enhancement tool.

Through an immense medical research study that was first reported in the *Journal of the American Medical Association* in 1989 (Blair, 1989), it was found that fitness levels are most effectively enhanced by regular, moderate, low-impact exercise. The study followed 13,344 people (10,224 men and 3,120 women, ages twenty to sixty) for eight years. This is 106,752 person years and almost 39 million person days.

Science is happiest when large numbers substantiate the relevance of the data. These are huge numbers. This study satisfied doctors and scientists that by simply becoming a little bit more active, advancing from sedentary to just mildly active, people improved their health. Another way of stating the findings of this historic study: moderate exercise reduces the risk of premature death from all causes, including heart disease, stroke, cancer, and diabetes. The major killer diseases are preventable with only gentle fitness practices.

In 1996 this study and many others like it provided enough evidence for the United States Surgeon General's Office to release a sweeping announcement that fitness practices as mild as walking, working in the garden, or even waxing the car can comprise a fitness program. The Chinese somehow knew this three thousand years ago. It was noted in the surgeon general's report that even several brief sessions of ten minutes are as good as one longer session of thirty minutes (DHHS, 1996).

Scientific studies have now confirmed ancient wisdom: low-intensity fitness methods are frequently preferable to more vigorous forms of exercise. Health benefits are still gained, while the risk of injury from more vigorous and intense practices is eliminated. This is a profound turning point in the history of health and fitness in the Western world. It suggests that the approaches to fitness from previous eras—such as pumping iron, jogging, high-impact aerobics, jazzercise—are not actually more effective in enhancing fitness levels than mild, low-impact fitness practices. Previously, fitness practice required athletic will and strength, but now anyone, even the very sick and the very weak, as well as average healthy people, can engage in health-enhancing and self-healing fitness practices.

The biggest surprise is that simple, mild exercise is actually a superior fitness practice. This is not to suggest that intense training is inappropriate for athletes. However, it is interesting to note that Olympic teams in Europe, Asia, and America have been including meditation and focused breathing in their training for a number of years. Mild practice is less likely to cause damage to bones, joints, tissue, or the immune system.

In the highly dynamic conventional fitness methods, the body mobilizes increased levels of internal resources but then spends them as fuel for hungry muscles. Milder fitness practices also mobilize greatly enhanced internal resources. However, instead of being rapidly consumed as fuel for the muscles, these potent resources flood the body. Like a cup running over, these resources, which comprise the medicine within, nourish and heal organs and glands to enhance health and heal diseased areas.

The methods of movement and the postures that you are about to learn may seem unusual when compared to the more familiar vigorous exercises like aerobics, calisthenics, running, and weight lifting. But our primary focus with these practices is to enhance the activity of the natural self-healing resources within. Movements and postures that appear to have minimal movement or activity are actually the most profound methods for generating, circulating, and conserving your own inner medicine.

When gentle movement is integrated with full relaxed breathing and deep relaxation of mind, the human body enters an especially healing and restorative state. This has a distinct effect on the blood, the nervous system, the immune system, the lymphatic system, and oxygen metabolism.

Honor the guidelines for mastering the self-applied health enhancement methods (SAHEM; see page 26). These movements are meant as a starting place for your own inventiveness. Please, do not sabotage your possibilities by thinking they must be done a certain way. Be innovative, and modify the practices to suit your needs, limits, and interests. Make the practice of self-healing fun.

Be careful; respect your limits. Balance and blend the breath and relaxation practices with the mild effort of the movements. This combination more dramatically mobilizes the vitality of healing resources within you.

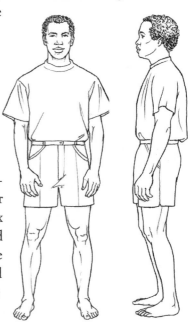

The Preliminary Posture

Start by standing with your feet directed forward at about shoulder width. Allow your shoulders to relax and arms to dangle at your sides. Bend your knees just slightly and allow the coccyx (tailbone), sacral bone, and pelvis to swing slightly underneath the spine. The lower back will adjust to be straighter and more elongated with less of a forward (lumbar) curve. It is not so much that you tuck the pelvis underneath as you would in ballet; rather you allow the pelvic bowl to adjust itself so that it is upright. Notice that the slight bend in the knees helps to allow the bowl of the pelvis to be upright.

If the lower back is curved forward, the bowl of the pelvis will tend to tip forward. The organs, which are like fruit within the bowl, will also spill forward. If the bowl of the pelvis is upright, then the fruit (the organs) rest within the bowl. Allow the spine to be upright. Adjust your head so that it is directly on top of your spine and shoulders; nod as if to say "yes"—this adjusts the chin gently downward, neither tucked nor rigid, and lengthens the back of the neck. Take a deep breath and relax.

This is called the preliminary posture and is an important health enhancement and self-healing practice in its own right. Many variations of the self-applied health enhancement methods from China actually use this standing method along with deep relaxation as a basic self-healing practice. It is called "standing meditation." Often the arms are adjusted to a position in front of the chest or face with the palms toward the body as if one were holding a large ball. In both hospital programs and public programs in the parks at dawn, individuals, small groups, and even very large groups do self-care practices that consist simply of standing in a deep state of meditation.

You can do the preliminary posture anywhere: while waiting for someone, standing in line, watching the sunset, or riding the bus. Relax deeply; imagine, or feel if you can, your internal energy circulating. Modify this preparatory position for sitting. People who work at a desk or use a wheelchair can use this same Preliminary Posture.

Application Suggestions

You can use this preparation for beginning most of the gentle movement practices in this section, or use it alone as a standing meditation. First, simply decide to initiate the Preliminary Posture. Just remembering to shift your posture in this way is a health enhancing practice that you can use anywhere. Once you have shifted to this position and reminded yourself of its value, take a few deep breaths. Then either return to your work, begin one of the gentle movements, or deeply relax into a meditation state. We will explore several forms of meditation in chapter 7.

Benefits

Just deciding to return yourself to this position has numerous benefits. You have to be aware enough to remember to do it. This awareness alone is empowering. You must relax enough to make the adjustments. This relaxation also has a health-enhancing potential. Simply shifting to this posture has an effect on brain chemistry because you have to relax to concentrate on arranging the body parts. Most people just keep on going through their day in body postures that are detrimental to health. The adjustment of the body to this Preliminary Posture optimizes the function of all organs and glands because it is the very posture in which they were designed to work well.

The Flowing Motion

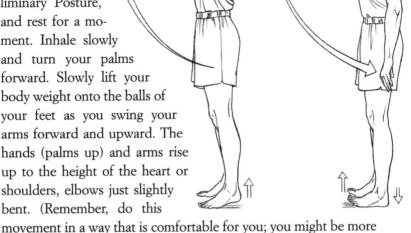

Arrange your-self in the Preliminary Posture, and rest for a moment. Inhale slowly and turn your palms forward. Slowly lift your body weight onto the balls of your feet as you swing your arms forward and upward. The hands (palms up) and arms rise up to the height of the heart or shoulders, elbows just slightly bent. (Remember, do this movement in a way that is comfortable for you; you might be more comfortable sitting.) Allow your mind to be free of concerns. Now, turn the palms downward, exhale, lower the arms slowly, and sink the body weight down so the feet are flat on the ground. When the hands pass the legs, allow them to continue to swing toward the back slightly. Lift your toes as high as possible.

Allow the breath to be full but not urgent. Deepen your relaxation. Turn the palms forward, begin to inhale, and repeat the movement. Build up a gentle rhythm. Soon, as you continue gently, you will gain a sense of ease, a flowing sensation. At both the top of the arm swing and at the back of the swing there is a smooth turn of the palm to change direction, a gentle rounding motion. If you feel unstable rising on the toes, then practice this method for some time with the feet flat on the ground. Eventually when you begin to do the heel and toe raises, this practice will help you to regain a sense of balance.

Notice that once you get the Flowing Motion going, you can rest in the rhythm and flow. It is almost as if the movement goes on its own and you can ride it. The Chinese believe that the human body exists in a "field" of energy. You may begin to feel as if you are floating within this field and to sense the flow of the energy as well as the circulation of the medicine within.

This is not a complex technique, but it easily mobilizes numerous health enhancement mechanisms in your body. For many in China this is a favorite exercise. The Chinese say, "Do this practice a thousand times each day and you will live forever." They also say, "Do this practice a hundred times a day and you will be healthy for a long life."

I have seen people doing this practice really quickly, even while walking along. They are probably trying to get their one thousand repetitions in each day and become immortal. Actually it is much more effective to do the Flowing Motion slowly. It is okay if your breath does not match the movements. In fact, advanced practitioners allow the breath and movement each to have its own rhythm.

Sitting and Lying-Down Variations

If it is necessary or desirable for you to do this practice while sitting, the instructions are essentially the same. While sitting, lift the heels and put the weight

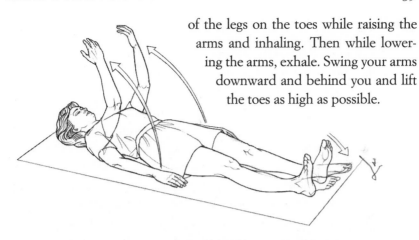

of the legs on the toes while raising the arms and inhaling. Then while lowering the arms, exhale. Swing your arms downward and behind you and lift the toes as high as possible.

This practice can also be modified to be done lying down in a hospital bed. Lift the arms and breathe in, lower the arms and exhale. Coordinate the foot movements, pressing the toes away from your head and then pulling them toward the head.

Variation for the Frail or Weak

If you or the individual whom you are working with is very weak, then adapt the method. Just lifting the fingers and pointing the toes will mildly enhance blood and lymph circulation and initiate a subtle restoration of strength and vitality. You may even simply imagine the movements. Research has demonstrated that the brain does not differentiate between an actual action and an imagined action. *The inner self-healing mechanism will be activated even if the movements are just mental images.* Simplify your thoughts, relax, and deepen the breath.

Application Suggestions

- *Health maintenance:* One session per day, ten to twenty repetitions, more if you wish.
- *Health improvement:* One or more sessions per day, twenty to fifty repetitions each time.
- *Disease intervention:* Start *slowly* and build up to two or more sessions per day, ten to twenty repetitions each.
- *Getting started:* One to three sessions per day with just a few repetitions.

Benefits

The movement in this practice requires gentle activity of many of the body's muscles. This demands an increased production of energy, which gently accelerates the blood's circulation of oxygen and nutrients. The oxygen, nutrition, and energy become available throughout the body as healing resources, aspects of the medicine within. The slow, relaxed pace reduces the constriction that the autonomic nervous system (the aspect of the nervous system that regulates organs) often causes in the blood vessels, so this lowers blood pressure. This in turn also increases the circulatory potential of oxygen and nutrients. In addition, the brainwave frequency is decreased into the alpha range, which is associated with numerous self-healing responses. And the deep breaths support relaxation.

The deep breaths also cause the diaphragm to descend and compress the lymph-rich tissues of the organs and glands. This propulsion of the lymph carries toxins out of the body, as well as carrying the immune cells throughout the system. The movement of the arms also pumps the lymph in the axillary area, which is where the arms meet the body. This is very helpful in circulating the lymph in the breast area in women. The contraction and relaxation of the muscles of the legs and feet pump the lymph from the lower body upward against the force of gravity and assists the flow of blood.

This is an excellent practice to help maintain or regain endurance in individuals who have become weak or balance in older people.

Right and Left Bending of the Spine

Beginning from the Preliminary Posture, bend the upper body gently to the right, exhaling. Allow the right arm to drop along the side of the right leg. Dangle the head toward the right shoulder. The left arm should drop gently across the front of the body, relaxed. Slowly return upright to center, inhaling. Then bend to the left, exhaling. Allow the left arm to drop down and the head to bend toward the left shoulder. The right arm will dangle across the front of the body. Inhale as you return to the upright position. Continue bending to both sides with relaxed, slow breaths.

The part of you that believes that things must be difficult and complex in order to be beneficial may complain, "This is too simple; how can an exercise so mild have any value?" If this is too easy, spread your feet apart and bend farther to the side. On the bending side, the lower hand may be propped against the upper leg for stability and to reduce strain. Allow the arm and hand on the stretching side to reach up over the head. This gives an even more effective stretch to the side of the body that is lengthening. Repeat slowly to both sides. Link the movements to deep, slow, relaxed breaths.

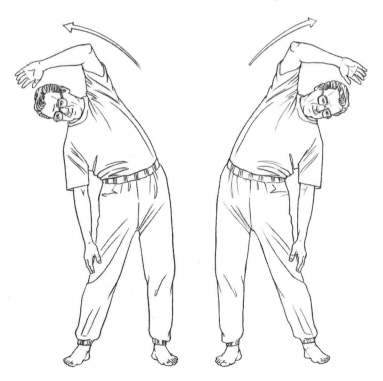

Sitting and Lying-Down Variations

If you are doing this in a chair or wheelchair, adapt either of the variations of this exercise as shown in the figure.

In bed or on the floor this practice can be adapted by reaching the right hand toward the right foot and bringing the right foot toward the head. Lift the left shoulder upward and extend the left foot away or downward. Then switch, moving the left hand toward the left foot and bringing the right shoulder upward. Pause between each movement, breathe deeply, relax.

Many of my patients have called the lying-down version of this movement their "special back exercise" because it has been remarkably beneficial for resolving pain in the back, ribs, neck, and shoulders. Doing this to both sides for a few minutes before falling asleep and for a few minutes after awakening is very effective, or it can be done anytime throughout the day. An alternative to doing this slowly is to speed up the shift from right to left so that you do four to five shifts with each inhalation and four to five with each exhalation.

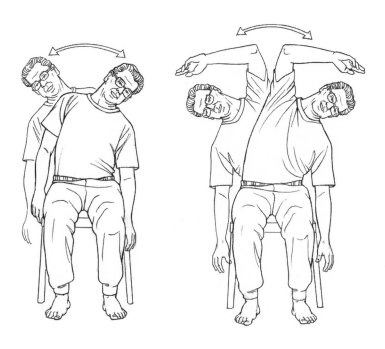

Application Suggestions

- *Health maintenance:* One session per day, five to ten repetitions.
- *Health improvement:* Two or more sessions per day, five to ten repetitions.
- *Disease intervention:* Start slowly and build up to three or more times per day, five to ten repetitions.
- *Getting started:* Just do the lying-down version several times in bed. Or do just a few repetitions standing or sitting.

Benefits

✦ This is an easy but extremely important exercise for the muscles along the spine, the neurological reflexes along the spine that activate the organs, and the connective tissue that holds the spine together. It is rare for people to exercise the flexibility of the spine in a side-to-side manner; this movement is excellent for maintaining side-to-side flexibility.

   Perhaps this makes you ask, "Why did the architect of the universe design the body and the spine so that they can bend to the side like this, since it is a movement that we rarely use?"

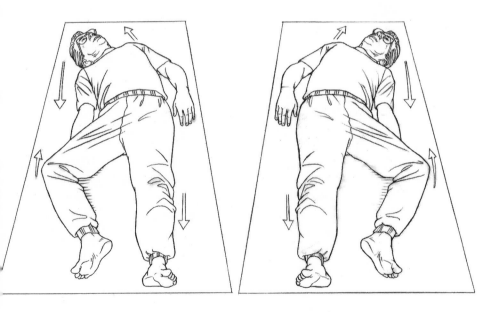

There are actually several rather profound reasons. The movement massages the contents of the intervertebral disks toward the center of the disk itself, which helps to sustain the bulk of the disk in spite of the downward pull of gravity. This is like fluffing the pillows between the vertebrae. Fluffing the disks also maintains a healthy distance between the vertebrae, which allows enough room for the exit of nerves from the spine that operate muscles and organs. When the disks collapse and this space thins, it causes pain and the malfunction of body movement or organ activity. This side-to-side massage complements the action of the next exercise, Front and Back Bending of the Spine.

In addition, this exercise alternately expands and compresses the sides of the rib cage, helping to increase or maintain the flexibility of the ribs and the capacity to expand the rib cage in breathing. The organs on the compressed side are squeezed, causing the propulsion of the lymph within them; this eliminates waste products, cleanses the tissues, and enhances the functioning of the organs.

The benefits of modified breathing and deep relaxation are present as well. It is true that this exercise seems very mild. However, these benefits have a subtle but powerful effect, enhancing the body's ability to sustain health, endurance, and comfort. Used over time it can make a significant difference in a wide array of functions because of the effect on the relationship between the spine and the organs.

Front and Back Bending of the Spine

Beginning from the Preliminary Posture, raise the hands upward, inhaling. The arms are bent at the elbow at approximately a ninety-degree angle. At first the palms of the hands face the body; as the arms raise, turn the palms to face downward at the level of the chest, forward at the level of the face, and then upward as the arms reach upward. The hands are opened with fingers outstretched but relaxed. The chest area stretches and opens. This is actually extremely simple, as the illustration shows.

When the arms come above the shoulders, the palms face upward, elbows still bent, as if holding up the sky. The head extends

upward on the spine and
tilts slightly backward. The
gaze is directed skyward,
between the hands, with
the eyes wide open. The
tailbone (coccyx) is tilted
backward. The curve of
the spine is like a bow
with the belly and chest
forward.

Then, on the exhalation,
the arms and elbows come forward and down, the palms turn
slowly toward the face. Clench
your hands into fists that close
tightly before your eyes; your eyes,
too, may be closed tightly. The elbows remain bent. The fists press together (hold them side to side or
face the knuckles together and
press) firmly in front of the chest.

Exert effort in the arms and chest muscles. The spine reverses to
bend the opposite way; the bow of the spine is now curved backward. The head is bent forward and the shoulders are rounded
forward. The tailbone is curved under and forward. The exhalation is full and somewhat forceful. Repeat the movement. On the
inhalation relax deeply, and allow your mind to seek freedom from
busyness, to be restful and calm. On the exhalation contract even
the eyes and the toes; everything contracts.

This practice is probably the most powerful lymph propulsion
method ever developed. It is also, obviously, quite mild. Feel free
to do multiple repetitions. It is simple, mobilizes the medicine
within, and causes no side effects. Build the number of repetitions slowly, and be sure to stay in your comfort zone.

With slight modifications this simple method becomes a powerful tool for increasing the flow of lymph in the breast tissue in
women and the prostate in men. Because of the absence of muscle in the breast area, there is no contraction mechanism in the

area for circulating the lymph. A number of studies have demonstrated that mild exercise reduces the risk of breast cancer (Bernstein, 1994). It has also been found that extreme fitness training actually increases breast cancer risk. This practice can be targeted at optimizing lymph flow in the region around the arms and torso. Bring the arms along the side of the body on the exhalation, and exert some pressure as the upper arms contact the rib cage. Maintain the pressure as the arms move forward along the sides of the rib cage. Compress the breast tissue between the arms as they move toward the front and the fists press together on the exhalation. At the end of the forward movement, gentle pressure is concentrated from above and below by the bending of the spine, which brings the shoulders toward the hips. Pressure is exerted, as well, from the sides by the arms. Continue on to the inhalation, and keep the upper arms together as they rise upward, giving a gentle lifting and compressing to the breast tissue before the elbows begin to part for the conclusion of the inhalation.

To enhance the pelvic organs you may extend the benefit of this practice by contracting the perineum (the same muscles that are used to restrain the flow of urine), which is located where the legs come together at the top, inside the base of the pelvis. This contraction is coordinated with the exhalation. It has been used both in China and in India for many centuries to circulate fluids and healing energy in the pelvic area. Traditionally, this is believed to have a special effect on the uterus and ovaries in women and on the prostate in men. More recently, this gesture has been recommended in Western medicine by gynecologists for women's pelvice health. It is recommended by urologists for men to sustain the health of the pelvic organs, strengthen urinary muscle control, and enhance sexuality. It is an excellent strategy for the prevention of prostate disorders.

Sitting and Lying-Down Variations

This practice can easily be done sitting in a chair or wheelchair, and it can also be modified by individuals who are confined to bed.

If emphysema or any other seriously debilitating disorder is a problem, be careful to build up to taking deeper breaths very slowly and gently over an extended period of time.

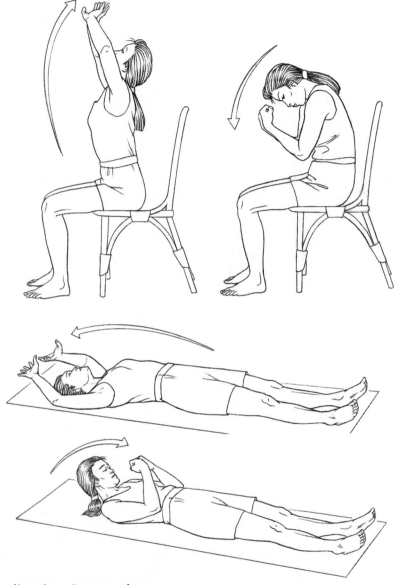

Application Suggestions

- ○ *Health maintenance:* One session per day, ten to fifteen repetitions.
- ○ *Health improvement:* Two or more sessions per day, ten to fifteen repetitions each time. Or fifteen to twenty repetitions in one session.
- ○ *Disease intervention:* Start slowly and build up to five or more sessions per day, ten to fifteen repetitions each time.

○ *Getting started:* Do five or six repetitions to begin to get a feel for the practice.

Benefits

The process of dramatically filling and emptying the lungs builds strength and endurance in the lungs themselves. The natural rib cage flexibility is utilized and maintained, or in those who have lost this flexibility, it is rehabilitated.

The action of the diaphragm in the large breaths, the bending motions, and the muscle contraction on the exhalation pump the lymph dramatically. The forward and backward flexibility of the spinal column is maintained, preventing the tendency to "slouch" or "stoop" forward. The disks between the vertebrae are massaged so that the material within them is concentrated toward the center. This complements the effect of the Right and Left Bending of the Spine. It ensures that there is enough room between the vertebrae to allow the nerves to carry information from the brain to the organs, glands, and muscles.

Because the mind is calm and free of concerns during this exercise, you gain the tremendous benefits of slowed brain-wave frequency and of the neurochemistry of relaxation. The contracting and releasing of the muscles of the hands and arms, the muscles around the eyes, and the muscles of the perineum further accelerate lymph flow and blood circulation in those areas. This increases the potential healing effects of nutrition and oxygen from the blood and the propelling of the by-products of metabolism into the elimination system by the lymph. The agents of the immune system are delivered to their targets more swiftly by the accelerated flow of the lymph. The coordination of the deep breathing and its large movement of the diaphragm with the total body contractions of the muscles creates a powerful lymph pump. Squeezing and releasing the tissues to move internal water is like plunging a dirty sponge into clean water and squeezing it over and over to remove waste and debris.

With special attention to contracting the perineum and to compressing the breast tissue with the arms, this exercise is partic-

ularly powerful as a tool for sustaining the health of the organs
that are the most vulnerable to disease in both men and women.
Using simple preventive methods to reduce the risk of breast and
prostate cancer is much better than waiting until the disease has
⊢ set in. In cases where breast or prostate cancer has been diagnosed, the opportunity for prevention has obviously passed. If you
have been diagnosed as having breast or prostate cancer, it is suggested that you confirm with a doctor knowledgeable about self-
care and lymph science that this movement is beneficial for you.

Reaching Upward, Stretching Outward

Begin with feet together or apart—your choice. As you inhale, lace
the fingers together and bring the palms, facing toward the body,
past the chest. As they pass before the face and eyes, rotate the
palms so that they are facing downward, then outward, and then
upward toward the sky. Extend the arms upward. Rise up on the

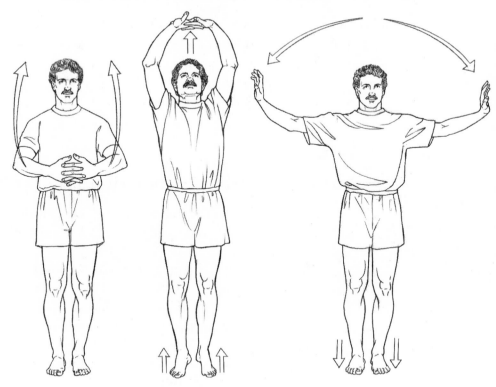

balls of the feet. Hold the position and the breath for a moment. This is called "Supporting Heaven," an ancient practice. Then unlace the fingers as the exhalation begins. Extend the arms outward to the sides. Point the tips of the fingers upward, aim the palms outward, and reach out from the center of the body to the heel of the palm as the arms are lowered. Lower the heels of your feet as well. Repeat slowly.

Find a rhythm for linking the movement and the breath that is deep, slow, and relaxed, or allow the breath and the movement to have separate rhythms. Either is fine. Focus your mind on something simple, and relax deeply. The movement is easy, and as you fall more and more deeply into relaxation, notice that the rhythm of the movement becomes somewhat hypnotic. It is almost as if the movement is doing itself, and you can just rest.

You may vary this movement by keeping the fingers locked at the top of the gesture and then bending forward at the waist until you are reaching down toward the ground. Bend gently, remembering to honor your comfort zone. Only bend over to the point where it is completely comfortable, no further. Over time your range will expand. Be patient, be gentle. Wiggle a little to release the spine. Then return to the upright posture, allowing the arms to dangle and unbending the spine, vertebra by vertebra, in a rolling motion. Rest for a moment and then repeat the motion.

Sitting and Lying-Down Variations

In the sitting position this exercise is nearly identical, including lifting up the heels.

In bed, link the fingers in front of the chest and then press upward from the sternum area. Hold the breath for only as long as is comfortable. Unlace the fingers, exhale while slowly lowering the arms to the sides. You may add movement with the toes as shown in the illustration.

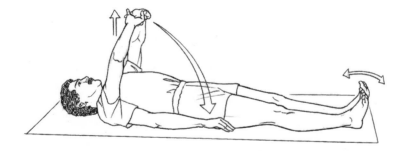

Application Suggestions

- *Health maintenance:* One session per day, five to ten repetitions.
- *Health improvement:* Two or more sessions per day, five to ten repetitions. Or do twenty repetitions in one session.
- *Disease intervention:* Start slowly and build up to several sessions, four to six repetitions each time.
- *Getting started:* In one to three sessions a day, do this practice once or twice slowly and carefully.

Benefits

The act of reaching up expands the rib cage, which increases lung capacity and strength. Rising up on the toes strengthens the lower leg, contributes to balance, and pumps the lymph from the lower limbs. The deep breath pumps the lymph fluid, particularly in the abdominal cavity when the diaphragm drops down. The process of exerting effort and then relaxing also propels the lymph. Relaxation during this practice expands the blood vessels, reducing blood pressure and allowing oxygen and nutrients to penetrate the tissues. In addition, relaxation increases the self-healing neurological functions that are active when the autonomic nervous system is at rest, promoting decreased brain-wave frequency and the production of healing neurotransmitters.

Spontaneous Movement Practice

Begin with the Preliminary Posture. Linger in this position, deepen the breath, and relax more and more deeply with each exhalation. From here begin to move about, guided by your

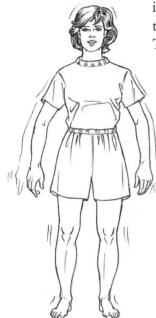

intuition or inner sense of what is needed. In China this is called Spontaneous Movement practice. There is no prescribed movement. The practice is based purely on your inner guidance.

In most kinds of group practice in the parks in China, everyone does certain movements together in unison. When groups do the Spontaneous Movement practice, each individual is doing something different. Some people are wiggling, some shake their arms, some are bouncing, some are flowing, some are doing self-massage, some are standing or sitting quietly, some are jumping about, some are making sounds. All are following the messages from within themselves, their inner wisdom. This is like listening to the healer within.

The Spontaneous Movement practice is a powerful tool for releasing emotional stress. The Chinese view the world and the universe as an immense but gentle chaos. This method is sometimes called "Dancing in Chaos." When the goal is to shake loose emotional tension it is helpful to move about dynamically and release deep sighs of relief. Spontaneous Movement is a particularly powerful method for accelerating the production of natural internal medicines because it is a direct response to inner guidance, and it so effectively helps to release emotional tension.

Allow yourself to wiggle, shake, bounce, flow, massage, stand, sit, jump, or produce sounds. Try the Sighs of Relief from page 92. Shake your hands, snap your fingers. Follow your inner guidance. This will seem awkward at first. However, it is actually the easiest practice because it is completely spontaneous and there is nothing to learn. Imagine you are attempting to work the medicine within into tight areas where it has not been able to reach. Imagine that you are working healing resources through areas that have been blocked or stuck. Focus on remaining relaxed, and allow the breaths to be deep and slow. After a while, stop and turn your attention inward; notice that you can literally feel the self-healing resources circulating within you. The sensation of the medicine within is particularly strong for most people after practicing this method.

This method is really fun to use with children. Their imaginations are free, and their inhibitions are few. It is a powerful tool to use with developmentally disabled or hyperactive children because it is so simple and it allows for the release of pent-up energy. This method helps to work out kinks in the morning before you get out of bed. Wiggle about, shift your position, wiggle your fingers and toes, rotate your ankles and wrists, yawn and sigh. Notice that this changes how you feel when you get up. In letters I receive after giving a lecture or teaching a class, people often comment on the Spontaneous Practice, because it is so easy to learn.

Application Suggestions

- ○ *Health maintenance:* Once a day for a few minutes.
- ○ *Health improvement:* Two times per day.
- ○ *Disease intervention:* Start carefully, and use this practice gently for a few moments several times throughout the day.
- ○ *Getting started:* Modify the practice. You might start simply by wiggling fingers and toes. Progress over time. Always make relaxation a key focus.

Benefits

On the days when this practice is vigorous, the benefits will be more directed at circulation of the blood and lymph systems. Particularly vigorous practice of Spontaneous Movement releases the connective tissue. On the days when it is more quiet and flowing, the benefits will be linked more to brain chemistry. Because relaxation will generally be mixed with the movement, Spontaneous Practice is an excellent way to produce what the Chinese call the Qigong (Chi Kung) state, where the maximum interaction of self-healing mechanisms is achieved. In this state, it is believed that the human system is especially able to draw from the healing energies of nature and the universe. Because this method is so easy to learn, so adaptable, and so effective for releasing emotional tension, it is a profound tool. In addictions to food, cigarettes, alcohol, and drugs it helps to release old patterns and produce healing neurotransmitters. It is very powerful for weight loss because the movement adjusts the metabolism and the tension relief reduces cravings. For cancer, AIDS, and other serious diseases it is particularly useful because it is so adaptable.

Simply moving the body is a powerful healing method. Recently, I met one of my favorite patients. He had originally come to the clinic for acupuncture for arthritis when he was eighty-two years old. He said, "The acupuncture helped a lot, but those exercises have really been great. I can't remember them exactly so I made up some of my own." I told him he looked really healthy. He said, "I'm going to be ninety-five years old this year. I wouldn't want to be ninety-five and not be healthy."

CHAPTER 5

Method 2
elf-Applied Massage

*The first healing gesture of the mother is to
reach out with soothing touch—massage. The
first healers of the human race, thousands of
years before the beginning of what we call
medicine, used hands-on healing—massage.
Massage is the most ancient healing art.*

John Harvey Kellogg,
physician, natural-healing pioneer,
Battle Creek Sanatorium

EVERY ANCIENT CULTURE ON THE PLANET EARTH HAS A
system of "hands-on" healing. What other medicine was there
thousands of years ago? Only herbs. In current times these practices are generally called *massage*. But there are actually many
systems in which the hands address the body in a healing way; they
include reflexology, medical massage, sports massage, connective
tissue manipulation, trigger-point therapy, zone therapy, pressure-
point therapy, acupressure (*tui na* in Chinese), and polarity.

As people begin to choose natural healing methods for their
health care, massage emerges as one of the primary therapeutic
modalities. Hospitals and even corporations are hiring massage
therapists to enhance health, help increase productivity, and

prevent the negative impacts of stress. Most of the newer comprehensive cancer treatment programs have begun to offer massage. Many forward-looking hospital systems have nurses on staff who practice "therapeutic touch," a special form of therapy using healing hands.

Several millennia ago Hippocrates, the father of Western medicine, relied on massage as a key tool for healing. Both ancient and current master physicians in the Asian cultures frequently make massage their primary healing specialty. Massage is available in every hospital in China. While it is particularly satisfying to receive massage from a trained professional or even a family member, it is possible and very effective to do it for yourself as well. The best part is that this can be done at any time of the day or night, no appointment is necessary, and there is no cost.

When a person is unwell or injured or when organ systems are malfunctioning, trigger points or pain reflexes appear throughout the body. Some of the points are directly in the area of the problem, while others appear at a distance from the problemand are known as reflexes. A reflex describes two separated areas that are in relationship in the body through the nervous system. Rubbing and exerting pressure on these points have been found over the centuries to have a positive effect on the healing process.

In some cases self-applied massage is very subtle; you may have to be patient and vigilantly apply the massage over a period of time. However, in many cases the results are dramatic. One of my patients is a piano teacher named Eileen. She had lots of students, and her services were in great demand. She attended and organized conferences, gave lectures, and was a judge at competitions. Over a number of years she found herself needing to urinate more and more frequently.

As the problem became more severe she began to experience terrible spasms of her bladder. She was forced to cut back on much of her professional life. She had to urinate four to five times during a one-hour piano lesson. She had to sit at the back of conferences so she could make multiple trips to the bathroom. The pain of the spasms began to keep her from traveling. Occasionally she would have to pull her car off the highway and lie on the seat until the pain subsided. Eventually she was forced to minimize her participation in most of her favorite activities.

I treated her with acupuncture, herbal formulas, and some body therapy at the Health Action Clinic. In addition, she learned to improve her health more quickly with the self-applied health enhancement methods. She immediately and enthusiastically began practicing breathing and relaxation techniques. Her self-care program included self-massage. She learned that if she could find and then rub the correct point in her ears, it could be of great benefit.

One day when she arrived at the clinic she announced, "Eureka, I found the point. When I rub certain ear points the pain scatters and the spasm subsides." With vigilant application of this and the other self-healing methods, she has been able to regain her health and return to her original lifestyle.

Medical massage has had significant research attention, and Chinese massage has had an immense amount of study reported in Chinese journals, but until recently, reflexology received little scientific attention. Alternative health care professionals who have been using reflexology had to just have faith that it is a relevant massage method.

Then, in 1993, a study was published in the *Journal of Obstetrics and Gynecology*. A strong control group and careful design gave this study a high level of credibility. Reflexology of the ears, hands, and feet was administered to patients with premenstrual syndrome (PMS). The patients receiving the therapy indicated a 62 percent reduction of symptoms (Oleson and Flocco, 1993). This is a new breakthrough in the ancient method of massage that has a reflex or distant effect.

Two Simple Approaches to Self-Massage

While there are many massage techniques, the self-healing approach to self-massage is purposefully simple. There are two primary notions involved in the practice.

First is the application of pressure and friction to points of the ears, hands, and feet that are reflexes to distant parts of the body. These reflex areas are called microsystems. A microsystem is an area of the body that is a small, local representation of the whole body. Thousands of years of experience have shown that the ears, hands, and feet are such areas. Each individual part of the whole human system has an associated reflex on the ear, on the hand, and on the foot. Typically, in the Western world this approach is called reflexology. Acupressure and shiatsu are the Asian pressure-point equivalents of reflexology. *Acupressure* is an English word for Chinese pressure-point massage; *shiatsu* is the Japanese word for the same concept.

Second is the application of kneading, stroking, pressure, friction, tapping, and gentle holding to specific areas of pain or dysfunction with the intention of having a local effect. In the reflex and acupressure systems, massage has its effect on a distant part of the body. When you massage with local intent, the aim is to affect the area that is being massaged.

Both of these systems tend to have an effect locally as well as by reflex, so there's no need to be confused. Just remember this simple rule: the greatest effect of massage will be gained from combining the benefits of treating the local area of concern with the benefits of treating the reflexes on the hands, feet, and ears. When self-massage is applied along with the other self-care techniques, you will experience a subtle renewal of health over time. Frequently the effect is quite dramatic.

All of the reflexes of the microsystems are linked through the brain and nervous system. During the first few hours of life, the whole body was a tiny embryo, just a few cells in size. The embryo carried within it the potential for a mature, full-sized self. As growth occurred, the extremities (hands, feet, and ears) carried the imprint of the whole system outward with them.

As the organ systems grew, they too carried the imprint of their relationship with the tiny original embryo. In the full-grown individual, the effects of this linking process are present in the reflex relationship of the microsystems in the extremities (ear, hand, foot) to all of the body's internal parts, organ systems, and functions. By stimulating the microsystems in the extremities, one stimulates by reflex the related parts and organs. Just above the lobe of the ear, in the middle of the big toe, and in the middle of the thumb are the reflexes for the brain, for example. In the Chinese system of energy flow it is believed that the distant effect is transmitted along the energy channels (see illustration on page 70).

With the application of massage aimed at a "local" response, the kneading, holding, pressure, friction, or tapping tends to accelerate the function of naturally occurring healing mechanisms in the area being massaged. This includes opening up the circulation of the blood, breaking up stagnant collections of lactic acid, bruised blood, and other metabolic waste products, propelling the lymph to flow more efficiently, and allowing for the arrival and departure of agents carried by the blood and lymph, such as immune cells, oxygen, enzymes, and other nutritional factors.

One of the best strategies for the reduction of the negative effects of stress or headache, for example, is to begin massaging the ear, hand, and foot reflexes as soon as you first sense the problem. To avoid jet lag, rub the reflexes every hour or so throughout the flight.

When insomnia is a problem, we have found that many people can change their sleep through self-applied massage. First, get out of bed and do a few minutes of one or two of the gentle movement practices from chapter 4. Then sit on the edge of the bed and massage the hands, feet, and ears. Finally, lie back in bed, take deep, slow, relaxed breaths, and run through one of the deep relaxation practices from chapter 7. We have had hundreds of reports from surprised insomnia sufferers who have stated that they don't remember finishing the deep relaxation.

To help quit smoking or to help curtail the use of alcohol or drugs, use a comprehensive program of self-applied health enhancement methods, but concentrate specifically on self-applied massage. The points you rub, particularly ear points, have been found to have a dramatic effect on brain chemistry. In addition, the simple act of rubbing the points occupies the hands.

Is it a coincidence that when you bend your arm at the elbow your hand automatically reaches your neck and your ears, ready to apply massage? Is it a coincidence that when you put your right foot on your left knee, your hands are right there to begin massaging? How far do you have to travel and how much does it cost to have your left hand massage your right hand? This is a health care breakthrough. Why have we overlooked this? Why didn't someone teach this to us as children?

Massage is the most ancient healing art and is a powerful healing tool. Our first impulse, when someone is experiencing pain and suffering, is to reach out and touch him or her in a helping way. This impulse was translated by the earliest humans into massage.

The self-application of this healing method is one of the oldest, most tried-and-true methods of self-care. With self-massage, your massage therapist is always with you. You can have massage almost anytime and almost anywhere—and it is absolutely free.

Massage Technique

Generally the massaging gesture, particularly of the foot, hand, and ear reflexes, is applied directly by thumb pressure or by kneading. It will take a while to build up your strength. This simple massage skill will serve you and others for your whole life. Alternate the thumb pressure with applications using bunched and extended fingers, the knuckles, the heel of the hand, or a gripping motion where the whole hand provides the force. Alternating the techniques gives your thumbs a chance to gain strength.

Start with light pressure and work up to substantial pressure. Imagine the pressure necessary to squeeze a new tennis ball or the strength necessary to pick up a brick between your thumb and the other fingers. These images will guide you on the amount of pressure necessary. If the pressure hurts the reflex, back off a bit. Notice that over a few days the amount of soreness will generally decrease.

The easiest guideline for self-massage is to find the sore points and work on them. To learn all about points and reflexes would be a lot. Such complexity would make self-massage hard to learn. This way it is easy and fun.

At the area of pain or dysfunction there are usually several (or one primary) painful or tender points. In the reflex microsystems of the hands, feet, and ears the sore points that you find are re-

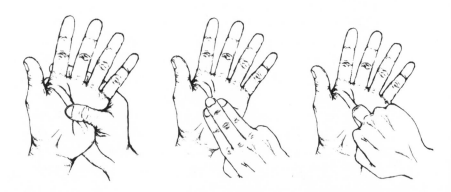

lated to distant areas. The earliest records of traditional Chinese medicine suggest that the original method for distinguishing the acupuncture points was to find sore points on the body. For example, imagine that you feel a headache coming on. First massage the hands, feet, and ears all over, looking for sore points. If you aren't in a situation in which rubbing the feet and ears is appropriate, then do the hands. Then come back and find the most sore points and concentrate on them. Next find the most tender points on the head, neck, and shoulders by massaging generally. Then come back to the most sore points and concentrate on them.

It is not necessary to know which sore point is related to which body part or function. Just follow the rule of finding the sore points and working on them. Keep it simple.

Massaging the Hands

The basic technique for self-applied massage of the hands is quite simple. The hands are so easy to reach. Without sitting down or

1. Heart (left hand) and thymus gland
2. Lungs
3. Liver (right hand) and shoulders
4. Solar plexus
5. Pancreas
6. Kidneys and adrenals
7. Stomach
8. Large intestine
9. Small intestine
10. Bladder
11. Appendix
12. Thyroid
13. Sacrum and pelvis

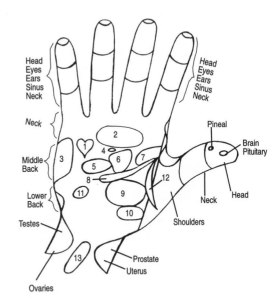

These points are from the Western reflex system. While certain organs like the diaphragm and the vagus nerve are not shown, they do have reflexes. Remember it is not so important to know much about such points and reflexes. Simply find the sore points and work on them.

having to remove any clothing you can go right to work. You can apply massage to your hands anywhere at any time.

You have probably seen the robes with large sleeves that the Chinese wear in pictures from ancient times. Often the person is shown with his or her hands held at about the level of the abdomen, tucked inside the sleeves. Not always but often these people are doing self-applied massage of the hands. There are certain ancient theories in Chinese medicine that link areas of the hands to particular organs and functions. This is similar to the reflexology concept, but the link is through the energy channels. For example, the application of thumb pressure to the palm from the heel near the wrist toward the little finger is thought to calm the heart and allow the mind to rest.

Self-applied massage of the hands can be very simple and far from esoteric. First massage your hands all over with firm thumb pressure. Notice areas of soreness and tenderness as you go. Then return to the tender areas and administer firm, kneading thumb pressure for a few minutes. Look for tender points on the back of the hands as well. Be sure to massage the fingers. Progress out toward the fingertips. Then, using the thumb and forefinger, press on both sides of the nail bed. These are special acupuncture points called entry and exit points. These tender areas are associated with body functions and organs that are not operating at their healthiest levels. Generally, if your health challenges are related to the upper part of the body, the tender reflexes will tend to be more toward the fingers, while health challenges from the lower part of the body will tend to be reflected in tenderness located toward the heel of the hand.

In numerous self-healing workshops over the years I have asked people to find the most tender area on their hand. Volunteers have, in turn, described their area of greatest sensitivity. Then, drawing on my best knowledge of the hand reflexes, I have advanced an "educated guess" as to what body area or function was their primary health problem. At several of these workshops a high percentage of correct "guesses" came from this seemingly primitive form of assessment. This was a surprise to everyone, including myself. These experiences certainly don't amount to scientific evidence, but they do encourage participants and inspire interest in the self-applied massage of the hand. When people simply find these sore spots and then work them over thoroughly on a daily basis, their health will improve.

Massaging the Feet

One of my earliest clinical revelations had to do with foot massage. After graduating from the study of Chinese medicine, I began my practice in Columbus, Ohio, with one of the first alternative

1. Head and brain
2. Pituitary and pineal glands
3. Throat and thyroid gland
4. Sinus
5. Eyes and ears
6. Shoulder
7. Heart
8. Lungs and thymus gland
9. Diaphragm and solar plexus
10. Stomach
11. Liver
12. Gall bladder
13. Kidney
14. Adrenal gland
15. Spleen
16. Pancreas
17. Small intestine
18. Large intestine
19. Bladder
20. Sacrum and sciatic nerve

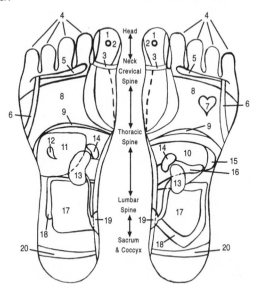

These points are from the Western reflex system. While certain organs like the bronchial tubes and the appendix are not shown, they do have reflexes. Remember it is not so important to know much about such points and reflexes. Simply find the sore points and work on them.

medicine and natural healing clinics in America. The Beechwold Clinic was started under the leadership of Dr. Ernest Shearer, an osteopath, in 1942. To find a holistic clinic in 1977 in Columbus, Ohio, was a revelation in itself.

Dr. Shearer offered me a position as a clinical associate on one condition: that I would provide foot reflexology treatments to patients each morning. He claimed that this would teach me a lesson I would never forget. Every patient of the clinic received foot reflexology every time he or she came in. This was the primary treatment for all disorders. Acupuncture, herbs, massage, osteopathic and chiropractic manipulation, colon cleansing, and other therapies were the secondary treatments, complementary to the reflexology.

I followed through on this morning practice for a little over eighteen months before I got so busy doing acupuncture that I had to change my schedule. In that time I administered foot massage during more than five thousand patient visits, totaling more than ten thousand individual feet. It was immediately clear to me that foot massage was effective. It was not unusual for people to exclaim that they felt better in a few moments.

I frequently taught the patients to use self-massage of the feet, hands, and ears at home. Dr. Shearer was right: I learned a lesson that I have never forgotten. It was a breakthrough to realize that reflexology was so powerful that it could be used effectively as a primary therapy. It is very effective when a doctor or therapist offers healing touch, especially when he or she also listens carefully to the patient's story. Even now, in my clinical practice of acupuncture and herbal medicine I tend to use massage much more than most of my colleagues. But most important, it became obvious to me that people could learn to perform this primary therapy on themselves and thus decrease their dependence on medicines and doctors.

The toes and ball of the foot are reflexes to the upper part of the body, head, eyes, sinuses, neck, and shoulders. The central area of the foot is a reflex for the torso, including the lungs, heart, and other internal organs. The heel is related to the parts of the body below the waist, including the sciatic nerve, hips, and pelvic organs.

Begin massage of the feet by applying pressure over the entire bottom of the foot. Usually the bottom of the foot is the primary focus; however, the top of the foot and the ankle area are rich with reflexes as well. Feel free to experiment in order to find the sore points. As you are massaging the whole foot, note the areas of particular tenderness. Come back and work specifically on the tender areas a second and even a third time. These are the reflexes that need it the most. Stimulating them and working out the soreness will affect the tissues, organs, and glands that are associated through the reflex mechanism, improving their ability to function.

Simultaneously you will be affecting the bones, muscles, nerves, and circulation of the foot itself. There are tools and devices available—foot rollers and tough rubber balls with raised areas—to assist with foot massage. They are helpful when reaching your own foot causes any strain. Even a kitchen rolling pin can be used: press the reflexes by rolling the foot over a rolling pin.

Massaging the Ears

The traditional systems of medicine from the Asian cultures have always included some type of massage stimulation to the ears. When you work on your ears, you will notice that within two to three minutes of vigorous massage your ears will get hot. This is caused by the increase of blood flow to the area. The Chinese say that when the blood is increased to an area, the healing energy is increased to that area as well. This increased energy to the ears is thought to stimulate the acupuncture reflexes, which in turn stimulate the related organs, tissues, and glands.

Notice that when you knead your ears for more than a few minutes they are extremely sensuous. This is because the ears are heavily laced with reflex nerve connections through the brain to all parts of the body. The presence of this high level of innervation is probably the reason why rubbing the ears is such a useful self-healing tool and why it feels so good.

Pressure on the reflexes stimulates heightened circulation of lymph, blood, and energy to the related areas of the body. In conventional Western physiology, we would attribute this to the circulation of blood and neurological impulses. The Chinese suggest that massaging the points in the ears actually enhances the circulation of the invisible vitality within, which they call the Qi (Chi).

1. Endocrine glands and hormones
2. Head and brain
3. Neck
4. Upper and middle back
5. Lower back
6. Heart and thymus gland
7. Lungs
8. Stomach
9. Small intestine
10. Large intestine
11. Spleen
12. Liver
13. Kidney
14. Bladder
15. Nervous system and spirit
16. Eyes and face
17. Shoulders
18. Arm and elbow
19. Hand
20. Leg and knee
21. Foot

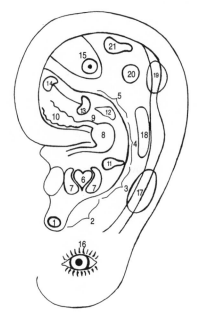

These points are from the Chinese acupuncture system. While certain organs like the pancreas and the prostate gland are not shown, they do have reflexes. Remember it is not so important to know much about such points and reflexes. Simply find the sore points and work on them.

It is amazing when you realize that simply bending your elbow brings your hand right to your ear, ready to massage. Is it possible that the architect of the universe had this in mind when designing the elbow? Why would we wait until we have lost our health and then drive across town to wait in a clinic in order to be medicated when a powerful self-healing gesture can be applied by simply bending the elbow and giving some massage to the ears?

A powerful case in point for the effectiveness of working with the reflexes in the ear microsystem is the use of acupuncture with points in the ears to treat addiction and weight loss. In innovative programs throughout the United States, ear acupuncture in conjunction with support group activity has demonstrated dramatic results. With the use of ear acupuncture, communities have found a reduction of over 50 percent in second arrests from drug- and alcohol-related offenses.

This is so dramatic, in fact, that most of the funding for these programs comes from the judicial system. Formerly, the treat- ment of choice for addictions was to use drugs to try to cure drug abuse—not a very congruent message. This may be the first time that money from the budgets of the police departments and the courts has been devoted to a health-based criminal rehabilitation program.

The acupuncture points for this treatment are all in the ears. I use this example because it is fascinating to note the extent to which treatment of the ear reflex points triggers powerful healing mechanisms in the human body. Research has shown that at least one way in which the stimulation of ear reflexes works is through the activity of the brain chemistry. Acupuncture or pressure stimu- lation of the ear reflexes stimulates the productivity of important neurotransmitters like endorphin, which is known to be a natural painkiller and an agent causing a sense of overall well-being.

One of our patients at the Health Action Clinic had an unusual pain that was caused by the contraction of muscles around his prostate gland. Sometimes this painful contraction would occur after sex. Occasionally it would occur spontaneously, without warning. It was very painful and would sometimes last for hours. He was against the use of medical drugs, arguing that they might relieve the symptoms but would not actually improve his health.

He tried relaxation, hot beverages, Yoga, and shifting to many different positions. He felt that acupuncture and herbal formulas were helpful in improving his health in general. What gave him the most direct relief of the intense pain in his prostate area, however, was self-applied massage of the ear. Within five to eight minutes of vigorous massage to the whole ear and about two minutes of massage to the prostate reflex, the pain would begin to disappear.

Massage of the ear is similar to massage of the foot and hand. Begin with moderate pressure and work over the entire ear on both the inside and the outside, using a kneading motion be- tween the thumb and forefinger. With the ears it is easy to do both sides simultaneously. Notice areas of discomfort. Return and work the uncomfortable areas vigorously. The lower part of the ear, the lobe, is related to the upper parts of the body—the head, brain, eyes, sinuses, and so on. The upper part of the ear is related to the lower parts of the body, including the lower back, hips, legs, and feet. The outer part of the ear, which you can knead between your thumb and fingers, is related to the muscles, bones, and joints. The inner part that is actually against the skull can be massaged by applying pressure from the extended index finger. This treats the internal organs and the glands. If your fingernail is too long, you can use the knuckle.

The ear is graphically represented in Chinese medical books as an inverted fetus. If you look carefully at someone's ear, you can imagine it as a baby curled up within the womb. The head is downward, and the arms and legs are curled upward with the feet and hands near the upper ear, in the fetal position.

This practice may not always bring the immediate results described in some of these examples, but vigilant application of self-applied ear massage over the long term, along with the other self-applied health enhancement methods, has helped many people to overcome serious health disorders.

Massaging the Neck and Shoulders

The neck and shoulders are often a starting place for back pain and headache. One of our best teachers about prevention is shoulder tension. If you keep your shoulders and neck free of tension, you will find it easier to think clearly and sustain high energy. Over the months and years you will become better able to catch tension early in its cycle.

Since it is always easier to prevent than to cure, you will have less to do to cure shoulder, neck, and head pain the earlier you take action to prevent it. Usually when tension starts to appear, we ignore it. Now, as tension begins to appear—apply massage. Remember to work on the hands, ears, and feet as a complement to massaging the local area. Use deep breathing and movement to enhance the massage. Use meditation to calm the nervous system and assist in prevention. When you have learned to prevent neck pain in this way, you will have learned how to prevent other health problems using the same methods.

There are many ways to approach neck and shoulder massage; here are several of the best. With your fingers together and extended, press in on the sides of the neck at the lowest point where the neck and shoulders meet. Press in on the right side and bend the head to the right, curving the neck around the fingers. Then press the other side and bend the head and neck to the left, curving around the fingers. Go slowly, exhale as you bend and press, inhale as you move to the next position.

Then move the fingers up about one inch on both sides and repeat. Bend and press right, bend and press left. Then move up again. Press right and left. Move up again and repeat. The distance between the shoulders and the head allows for four to five bends in each direction. Next, carefully speed the process up. Now it is as if you are gently tossing your head right and left. Allow the breath to flow naturally. Find the sorest or lumpiest spots all along the sides of the neck and work them thoroughly.

Next, lay the open hand over the back of the neck, palm against the spine. The right hand will lie with the fingers extending to the left side of the neck. Curl the fingers of the right hand to massage the left side of the neck. Press in, seeking soreness and tight areas. Then bend the neck left so that the weight of the head pulls to the left and the strength of the fingers pulls to the right, deepening the reach of the massage on the left side. Take a deep breath.

Shift to the other side. The left hand lies across the back of the neck, and the fingers of the left hand curl to apply pressure to the right side of the neck. Alternating pressure from the different fingers, seek sore spots and lumps. Try different breathing rhythms. Then lean the head to the right and pull the hand to the left, deepening the penetration of the pressure. Breathe.

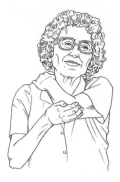

Now move on to the shoulders. Again, the right hand will work on the left side, but now your reach is across the front of the body. Throw the right hand around the front of your chest and reach as far over your left shoulder as possible. Start rubbing with curled fingers vigorously. Work the whole area, then go back and give special attention to the sore and tight areas. It may help to use your left hand to lift your right elbow; this will assist you in reaching further back. It also helps to lift and drop the shoulder that you are massaging to vary the pressure and to target areas of need. Also, move your torso about; this spreads the effect to the spine, ribs, and chest area. Sometimes the actual cause of shoulder, neck, or head pain is actually in the ribs, the chest, or the spine.

Now switch. Throw the left hand around the front of your body and over the right shoulder as far as you can. Begin massaging. Hold the left elbow up with the right hand if it helps to support your reach. Wiggle your torso, lift and drop your right shoulder. Try using the Sigh of Relief on the exhalations (page 92).

Tracing the Acupuncture Energy Channels

In the traditional Chinese healing system, it is believed that vitality or energy (Qi) circulates in the human body to sustain health and coordinate the function of the organs. The channels for the flow of this healing energy travel up the front of the body and down the back. When you do the Tracing the Channels practice, you may lightly stroke the surface of the body, or you may pass the hands an inch or so above the surface of the skin. The energy, it is believed by the Chinese and many Western scientists, is not contained inside the body but actually resonates in and around the body like a magnetic field.

Start by rubbing your hands together until they feel warm. Then, as if you were washing your face, pass your hands upward—starting at the neck and chin and then over the cheeks, eyes, and forehead. Pass your hands over the top of the head, down the back of the neck, and along the shoulders as if you were bathing in a powerful healing resource. Bring the hands around the front of the shoulders, under the arms and reach around the back and up as high on the back as possible. Continue down the back, over the sacrum, and down the backs of the legs.

As you bend over, be careful to notice where your comfort zone ends, and do not bend too far. If it is uncomfortable to bend forward, don't. Over time this method of gentle movement and energy massage will help the comfort zone to expand.

Come around to the front and inside of the legs and pass the hands upward. If you can comfortably reach your feet, then come from the back of the legs around the toes and up the front and inside of the legs. Imagine that you are standing in a pool of healing waters. As your hands come around to the front and inside of the legs, imagine that you are gathering from the pool handfuls of a

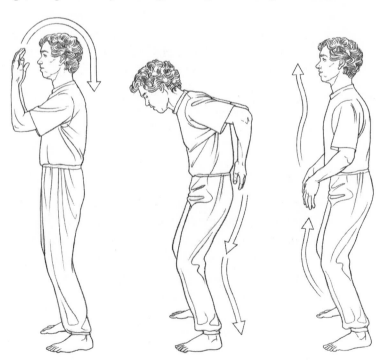

marvelous healing elixir. Bathe the front of your body, passing over the knees and thighs, pelvis, abdomen, and chest.

Linger in front of your heart for a few moments and rub your hands together again. Allow your breath to be full but not urgent, and drift deeper and deeper into relaxation. Free the mind from life's details. Feel the medicine within you circulating, or visualize water flowing, butterflies at play, or clouds sailing across the sky. Then begin again, a second cycle, bathing in energy, first the neck and face, over the top, all the way down the back. Gather the healing water as you bathe up the front. Linger for a moment in front of the heart while rubbing the hands together.

After you have done several rounds, down the back and up the front, and after you rub your hands together, take a moment with the palms of the hands facing each other. Feel the energy between your hands. In this deep state of relaxation, after stroking the energy channels, your energy is optimal and your mind is quiet. See if you can perceive a sense of fluff or magnetism between your hands as you move them together and apart slowly. Relax; it is not important to have this skill. The life energy is there, or you would not be alive. Give yourself lots of time to explore this energy; it is very subtle, and while some people feel it right away, for others it can take years. It is not necessary to feel the energy sensation to benefit from this self-healing method.

This method can easily be adapted for sitting practice. It is one of the most ancient Qigong methods. Repeat several cycles and then, if you wish, transition to the next method.

Massaging the Abdomen

When you reach the level just below the breast bone (sternum)—or if you are beginning, start in the Preliminary Posture—place one hand over the other and begin a circular motion following the pathway of the colon. The motion is clockwise, with the clock lying on your navel facing away from your body. Rub either with gentle friction on the skin or about an inch above the surface of the body. Starting from the point below the breastbone, pass the hands to the edge of the rib cage on your left, then pass the hands downward to the corner of the pelvis on the left; pass the hands across the pubic bone moving to the right to the corner of the pelvis, and then pass the hands upward to the corner of the rib cage on the right. Finish the cycle by returning the hands to the center below the breastbone.

Repeat this as many times as you wish. If your aim is to improve bowel function, resolve gastrointestinal problems, or enhance the function of the abdominal organs, do multiple cycles of this massage.

One of the most ancient and effective forms of massage from China is to find areas of tension in the abdomen and massage to release knots and lumps. Press inward under the sternum with your extended fingers held together; bend forward gently and press in. Press both directly in and under the bone, directing penetrating pressure toward the colon and other organs. Straighten back up. Shift the position of the fingers to the point halfway to the left corner of the rib cage. Press in, bend over, penetrate in and under the ribs. Return to the upright position. Move your fingers all the way to the left corner of the rib cage and repeat. Repeat this process at each of the twelve points noted on the illustration like the numbers on a clock. In addition, apply similar pressure to points nearer the navel.

Look for areas of pain, tightness, or lumpiness. This type of massage is a particularly healing method because it can remove accumulated tension from the abdominal organs and from the energy system in the abdominal area. A dozen of the most important energy channels travel through this area. You may repeat this several times in a session or several times in a day. It can be done while seated and even while seated on the toilet.

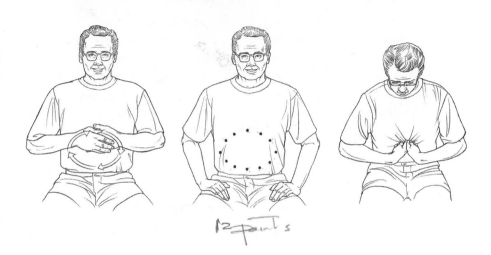

12 points

Some people like to inhale as they bend forward, others like to inhale as they return to the upright position—you choose. Pay attention to what you are experiencing. If you genuinely relax, the benefits of this process are accelerated substantially. To finish, repeat the circular movement of passing the hands clockwise several more times. Then, if you wish, you can proceed to the next method.

There are some who suggest that if the individual is experiencing diarrhea, the massage should go in the opposite direction for the hands-circling movement and the pressure method. Because there are many causes for loose bowels, I have found that most people benefit from the practice following the natural direction of material in the colon. This is particularly effective for weight loss. However, as usual, I urge you to pay attention and try both approaches to become an expert in your own situation.

Energizing the Organs

Place the hands over the lower edge of the ribs, near the sides of the body but still on the front. Beneath the right hand is the region of the liver, the gall bladder, and the upper right-hand corner of the large intestine. Beneath the left hand are the spleen, the pancreas, the stomach, and the upper left-hand corner of the large intestine.

Rub the open palm against the surface of the body in a circular motion. Notice that eventually you begin to feel warmth or even a tingling sensation. Then hold your hands still and feel the warmth penetrating the surface of the body and migrating to the organs. Allow the breath to be full but not urgent, and drift deeper into relaxation on each exhalation.

Think for a moment about these organs. They have served you faithfully for your entire life without ever having to be asked. Allow yourself to marvel at this and even smile quietly within as you acknowledge the service of these organs to you. Particularly on the exhalation, send the effect of this smile to the organs and perhaps send a wave of gratitude to them. Imagine that they are delighted to have your appreciation. Linger, sending warmth and gratitude to the organs for as long as it feels right. Don't rush.

Then move the hands so that one lies over the breastbone (sternum) and the other lies over the navel. Again, rub in a circular motion. Build up warmth. Then stop and hold the open hands still. Feel the warmth penetrating the surface of the body and radiating into the tissues. Under the upper hand are the heart, the thymus gland, and the lungs. These organs have never needed any instruction or encouragement; they just work for you constantly, loyally, vigilantly—the lungs transferring oxygen to the blood, the heart pumping oxygen and nutrition to the tissues, and the thymus creating an army of immune cells that protect you from the invasion of pathogens such as a virus, bacteria, or fungus.

Take a moment to be thankful. Use the exhalations to send a wave of gratitude to the organs along with a smile of wonder at the miracle of their unwavering service. Without them you would not be alive. Shift your attention to the navel. This was the prenatal passageway for all that nourished your growth in the womb. The Chinese conceive that after birth (postnatal), the body stores and circulates a special prenatal energy that is a primary component of the medicine within, the inner elixir. Subtle connections to this area remain intact from all parts of the body. Send a smile of gratitude through the navel and let it diffuse throughout your whole body. Linger until you feel that the effect of this gesture is complete.

Now move your hands around to the lower back. Keeping the palms open and against the surface, move your hands as high on the back as is comfortable. This is the area of the kidneys. The kidney organ is up under the ribs, but the acupuncture point for the kidneys is lower down, halfway between the ribs and the hip bones (pelvis). Rub the hands against the surface of your back to build up some heat. Then, allow the warmth to penetrate through

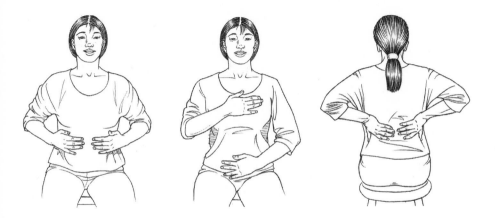

the surface of the skin toward the kidney energy points, especially on the exhalations.

In the Chinese tradition, the kidneys, in addition to eliminating waste, are (along with the adrenal glands that rest above them) the dwelling place of the essential life energies. In the Western tradition we do not yet understand well this association of the kidneys with vital energy. Nevertheless, in both traditions the kidneys are tireless servants of life and health. Along with the warmth from your hands, send a wave of gratitude for the kidneys' reliable service. Allow the inner benefit of your smile of appreciation to travel to the kidneys and the adrenals. Imagine their delight at having received your acknowledgment after all these years.

Complete the practice by bringing both hands to the front and resting them on the belly just below the navel. Remain for a moment longer in a state of deep rest. Allow the mind to be free and tranquil. The Chinese call this area the "elixir field." This means, literally, "the place within which the most profound medicine is produced and stored."

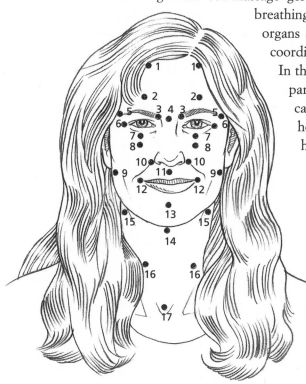

Following these self-massage gestures, along with focused breathing and deep relaxation, your organs and glands are in a highly coordinated and energized state. In this state the healer within is particularly active, and your capacity to produce internal healing resources is at its highest.

Massaging the Face and Eyes

There are many energy points on the face and around the eyes. These points are associated through the energy channels to the stomach, spleen, large intestine, lungs, small intestine, heart, bladder, kidney, and endocrine system. These acupuncture points can be treated with self-massage. The direct benefit is a healthy face and eyes; the indirect benefit includes healthy organs and metabolism. Keeping the internal organs healthy keeps the face and eyes radiant; keeping the face and eyes healthy contributes to sustaining health in the organs.

Massage of the points around the eyes is common in the schools in China, where children take breaks to do health enhancement practices that include self-massage. The massage of the eyes and face can be combined. Begin by working on the face points. You can tap the points sharply with the tip of your index or second finger. Or you may wish to give some gentle pressure with a circular motion, using two or three extended fingers held together. Notice that the tapping provides a bit more rousing sensation. After a session of facial massage you will feel a tingling that actually affects the organs as well as the facial area.

Spend a few moments on each of these areas. Feel free to add others or to linger at certain points longer. All of the points have a positive effect on the muscles and skin of the face, as well as the organ or channel they are associated with. The following list notes additional benefits according to traditional Chinese medicine:

1 Gall bladder point: Affects forehead lines, emotional tension, headache, addictions, the liver
2 Gall bladder point: Same as number 1
3 Bladder point: Affects bunch lines between eyebrows, eyestrain, headache, sinus; decreases water retention
4 Endocrine: Affects bunch lines between eyebrows, headache, eyestrain, pineal, pituitary; increases energy; facilitates weight loss
5 Endocrine: Affects crow's-feet at eyes, headache, eyestrain, brain
6 Gall bladder: Affects crow's-feet at eyes, emotional tension, headache, eyestrain, addictions
7 Stomach: Decreases puffiness under eyes, dark circles, affects digestion, the spleen; facilitates weight loss
8 Stomach: Same as number 7
9 Stomach: Firms skin, reduces jaw tension, affects spleen
10 Large intestine: Affects upper smile line at nose, sinus, lungs, elimination, and weight loss
11 Governing vessel: Affects the whole face; connected to brain

12 Stomach: Affects smile line at mouth, digestion, spleen

13 Conception vessel: Affects the whole face; related to life-source energy

14 Conception vessel and chin: Affects the tone of the skin, muscles, and glands of the chin; accelerates circulation of blood and lymph

15 Tapping and jiggling of throat and neck: Affects skin and muscle tone; accelerates circulation of blood and lymph

16 Endocrine: Drains lymph (from below the ear, tap and pull downward)

17 Conception vessel: Affects neck, particularly thyroid, which enhances metabolism and the vital energy of the whole system

To give additional attention to the eyes and eyesight go back and treat the points around the eyes: 2, 3, 4, 5, 6, 7. You may tap between these points as well—for example, all along the eyebrow from point 3 to point 5. Then rub the hands together to produce heat. Place the palms over the eyes so that all light is blocked out. Relax deeply, exhale, feel the warmth penetrating the eyes. Feel the heat penetrating back through the optic nerve to the part of the brain where sight occurs.

If you wish, while your eyes are closed, move them in a circle: look left, up, right, and down for several cycles. Then reverse: look right, up, left, and down for several cycles. Then squeeze your eyelids together tightly. If you pay attention, you may feel fluid pressing out of the area, like water being expressed by a sponge. Then uncover your eyes and open them with several exaggerated blinks. Look at something up close. See it carefully in detail. Then look at something far away; stay relaxed, don't strain. Look close again,

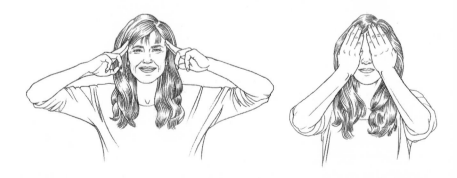

then look far. You may repeat this eye process several times. A number of people have used this practice successfully to improve their eyesight.

Massaging Reflexes First, Then Finding the Pain

This is one of the simplest methods for self-massage, and it is useful in nearly all cases. No matter whether your focus is pain relief, metabolic rehabilitation, or general performance enhancement, this technique is effective.

Start with a general focus on the three primary reflex areas—the hands, ears, and feet. After general massage of the reflex areas, then focus on the sorest spots in each of these areas. Remember, it is not so important to know what the sore areas represent or the cause of their soreness. The fact that they are tender to pressure indicates that they are linked to pain or dysfunction. The act of massaging these sore points promises improvement.

Following both general and specific massage of the reflex areas, the next step is to massage thoroughly the specific area of pain or dysfunction. For example, if you have shoulder pain, first massage the hands generally, seeking the sore spots, then return and give extra massage to the tender areas. Then massage the ears generally and return to give extra attention to sore points. Then do the feet, first generally, then the specific sore points. Now, go to the shoulders and give thorough massage to the local areas of discomfort.

If you are experiencing stomach or bowel trouble, use the same technique. Do general and then specific massage of the reflexes in the hands, ears, and feet. Then do local area massage on the stomach and bowels, using the methods of abdominal massage and energizing the organs. For headaches, do the reflex areas, then work directly on the head and neck. Because headaches are frequently a symptom of disharmony in the organ systems, reflex massage is actually more important than the massage of the local area of the head.

For health challenges like immune dysfunction, elevated blood pressure, anxiety, obesity, or insomnia, there is no local area to massage. The immune system is active throughout the body, and the circulatory system is active everywhere as well.

Finding and massaging reflex points (these are the same as acupuncture points) is particularly effective in healing these health challenges that do not have a specific location in the body. General practice of gentle movement, breathing practices, and meditation enhance the effect of the massage.

It is always easier to use massage as a preventive measure than as a cure after a problem has started. Use this massage method while you are well. Teach it to children. It is easy to remember. Just think: hands, ears, feet, followed by thorough massage of the part of the body that needs healing.

Connecting the Spots, Then Wiggling

This is another method that is quite effective and easy to remember. Start by rubbing your hands together to build up heat. Place one hand on the area of your body that is experiencing the greatest pain or tension. Place your other hand on another part of your body that experiences pain or tension. Then move about gently as in the Spontaneous Movement practice on page 51. Add Sighs of Relief (page 92) to release tension and emotional stress, and to accelerate the activity of the medicines produced within.

The theory for this method comes from Chinese medicine. Pain is caused by stagnant energy. When you place your hands over different parts of the body, particularly if you rub them together first to build up the healing energy (Qi), it stimulates circulation of the energy system within. The pathway of Qi circulation between the two hands helps to move healing energy through areas of Qi stagnation. The shaking and wiggling movements of the Spontaneous Practice accelerate the movement of the energy. Deep, relaxed breaths and voice sounds help as well.

In this self-massage method, several actions get the healing resources moving. It is like a symphony of interacting self-healing factors—movement, massage, and breath. Bring these together along with deep relaxation and you have activated all four of the self-healing methods at once.

Try placing your hands in several different positions. Press into lumps and tight places with extended fingers or thumbs. Rub with the palm of the hand to create additional heat. The tremendous benefit of this practice comes from moving the body in different directions than usual and then adding massage, focused breathing, voice sounds, and deep relaxation.

Application Suggestions

- o *Health maintenance:* one session per day of five to fifteen minutes for both hands and ears. Add the feet whenever possible. Always massage the local areas as needed.
- o *Health improvement:* A longer single session, or two sessions per day; try to include the feet for extra benefit. Add massage of the local areas.
- o *Disease intervention:* Start *slowly* and build up to frequent applications. Practice will increase the strength of your hands, and strength will allow deeper pressure and greater effect.
- o *Getting started:* Do brief sessions as often as possible. Be careful to honor the comfort zone.

Benefits

The practice of self-applied massage stimulates numerous physiological mechanisms that cooperate to enhance our natural self-healing capability. The explanation for reflex massage generally agreed on points to the fact that neurological impulses are transmitted from the reflex point on the surface of the body to distant sites by way of the nervous system through the spine and brain.

The benefits of massage to the local area include increased circulation of oxygen and nutrition and enhanced elimination of metabolic waste products in the lymph. Relaxing and deepening the breath during self-massage shifts brain chemistry and brain-wave frequency, which produces a healing mix of neurotransmitters and hormones. The massage itself also contributes to shifting the body chemistry toward the self-healing mode.

Pain relief is only one benefit of self-applied massage. It also stimulates balanced organ function. Metabolic disorders like diabetes, chronic fatigue syndrome, fibromyalgia, obesity, and even depression and anxiety respond to massage. It can help to clear the mind, enhance sleep, and reduce numerous symptoms of more serious diseases like cancer, HIV/AIDS, and multiple sclerosis. Massage is a powerful tool in gaining vitality following hospitalization and in rehabilitation of health following heart disease, strokes, and surgery. In most of the ancient medical systems massage was the primary healing art, and in China and India it was believed to refine and enhance the body's vital energy, the most subtle self-healing resource.

CHAPTER 6

Method 3
Breathing Practices

*Whoever can swallow the breath
like the tortoise
or pull the breath in and circulate it
like the tiger
or guide and refine the breath
like the dragon,
shall live a long and healthy life.*

Master Ge Heng,
alchemist and immortal,
second-century China

IT IS A BIT UNUSUAL FOR US IN THE WESTERN WORLD TO consider breathing techniques important. After all, we are always breathing, aren't we? It seems a little silly to give extra attention to something we do naturally, which is already working. But take a moment to notice your own breathing. Isn't each breath actually quite shallow?

Without moving or adjusting your position, take a really deep breath. Does your posture or position encourage or restrict your ability to take in full breaths? If you pay careful attention over time, you will probably realize that you are generally utilizing one quarter or less of your lung capacity. Notice also that to take a really deep breath you have to actually change your position.

There are numerous beneficial physiological mechanisms that are triggered when we turn our attention to the breath. When attention to the breath and breath rhythm is altered, dramatic physiological and even emotional changes can occur. Science didn't understand this until quite recently, but it turns out that the interaction of the lungs, diaphragm, and rib cage is a primary pump for the lymph fluid. This mechanism may actually be more important to lymph propulsion than muscle contraction and body movement, which are the generally accepted mechanisms for propelling the lymph fluid. Together the breath, body movement, muscle contraction, and several other associated physiological activities create a "lymph heart."

You can live for weeks without food and for days without water, but you can live for only moments without breathing. The breath is the source of oxygen, which is the key element in the body's ability to produce energy. Cells, particularly those in the brain, begin to die when they go without oxygen for even a few minutes. In addition, the act of relaxed, full breathing shifts the function of the autonomic nervous system toward a state of balance, which is called homeostasis. It is remarkable how many naturally occurring health restorative mechanisms are triggered or enhanced by the breath when we attend to it consciously.

Most ancient cultures emphasize special breathing practices. This has generally been considered strange and mysterious by Western researchers. Why would these cultures continue to employ such techniques for thousands of years? Empirical science—the scientific method of all original cultures—is based on trial and error. When something is found to have value, it is kept and employed. When something is found to have little or no value, it is dropped. In the empirical approach, the things that are kept are "tried and true." Empirically, breath practice is "tried and true."

Clinical experience also points to the value of breathing practices. Patients who have learned and used breath practice as a part of their daily personal system of self-applied health enhancement respond more quickly to treatment, no matter what type of physician they are seeing. Individuals who are well are able to sustain wellness, can adapt to greater stress, and have greater endurance when they keep breath practice in their daily self-care ritual.

Breathing practices are particularly applicable in the hospital or at the dentist's office. Alone or linked with the other self-applied health enhancement methods, the breathing practices accelerate the natural healing mechanisms in the body. When people are in a medical situation, they typically feel very much out of control or under the control of others. Using these breathing practices can give one a sense of control. One of the members of our Wednesday Self-Healing Practice Sessions found herself unexpectedly in the hospital for a second heart bypass. Her first bypass had been successful, but the experience had been terrifying. She says that the self-healing methods, particularly the breathing practices, helped her to feel like she was in charge of her situation. By using the self-healing practices along with prayer, she was able to transform the second bypass into a far less terrifying experience.

The word *inspiration,* which means literally "to breathe in," also refers to the rush that we feel when overtaken by spiritual energy. Inspiration is what we call the force that impels us forward into life with enthusiasm; it is the divine influence that brings forth creativity and vitality. The breath is a powerful link to the most profound medicine that we produce within us physically, mentally, and even spiritually.

We enact this nearly unconscious gesture, the breath, between 500 million and 630 million times in our life span (500 to 630 million breaths during seventy to ninety years of life). How inspiring to realize that this powerful healing tool is within us, just waiting to be used to its fullest capacity. Have you taken a deep breath yet?

You can take a deep breath in secret, in a meeting, in your car, while reading a book, at the theater, at work, on the phone, before you arise, before you sleep, during a conversation, while you bathe, during sex, at the bank, before or during any action. You can deepen your breath to interrupt a negative thought. Even our grandmothers' wisdom says, "When you are angry, breathe deeply and count to ten before you act."

You can take one or more deep breaths anywhere, anytime; no one will even know. Deepening the breath is the most flexible self-healing and health enhancement method. Remember the physicist, Bob, who discovered 107 activities throughout his day that would help him recall that it was time to take a deep breath. Unlike body movement, massage, or meditation, which require an obvious departure from normal activities, the deep breath can be done at the same time as you are doing almost anything.

Many people believe that deep breathing will increase the amount of oxygen in the blood. Frequently, teachers of Yoga and other health enhancement methods will say, "Take a deep breath, fill your lungs, and just load the blood with healing oxygen." Actually, this is not what happens. Even in people with lung disorders, the blood is generally more than 95 percent infused with oxygen when it leaves the lungs. With deep breathing or shallow breathing, there is plenty of oxygen in the blood.

Deepening the breath does not directly help send the oxygen in our blood into the tissues either. Oxygen migrates from the blood to the tissues because of oxygen demand, which is only minimally affected by the depth of the breath. However, when you take a deep breath, it does initiate relaxation. This causes the blood capillaries to expand, which allows a greater volume of oxygen to migrate to sites where healing is needed.

So, scientists have wondered: "If focusing on the breath doesn't increase the oxygen in the blood or release the oxygen into the tissues, then why is deep breathing so important?" In fact, the deep breath accelerates several other profound self-healing mechanisms. It pumps the lymphatic fluid, triggers relaxation, and initiates the release of numerous neuropeptides from the breath center in the brain. These are each powerful healers.

Your breath is always with you; you cannot separate yourself from your breath, except by giving up your life. Our first act when we emerge from the womb is to inspire. Our last act in life is to "dis-inspire," or expire. These breaths, first in and finally out, are like bookends. In between lie the chapters and pages in the books of our lives. It is no surprise that the breath is so remarkably linked to the power of healing.

The Essential Breath

This breath practice is the basis of most health enhancement breathing methods. It is the natural breathing pattern of the newborn baby. It is known simply as the abdominal breath. Many people have learned it as the "Yoga Breath."

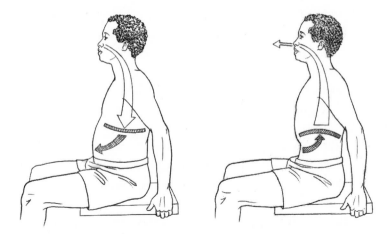

It is typical for people to become accustomed to breathing in a shallow way. While our typical breathing allows for survival, it does not increase vitality or accelerate healing.

First, adjust your posture so that your lungs, as well as your chest and abdomen, can expand freely. This is best accomplished by standing or sitting erect. You may also do this practice lying down. Breathe in through the nose, filling the lower portion of the lungs first. This will cause your abdomen to expand as the diaphragm drops down and compresses the internal organs. Then allow the upper lobes of the lungs to fill. This expands the ribs and chest cavity. You will feel a tremendous sense of satisfaction when your lungs are completely full.

Then exhale slowly through the nose. Repeat. When the Essential Breath is done optimally, you will reach the point of fullness, naturally rest for an instant, and then spill over a threshold into a long, slow exhalation. When you take a slow, full breath and reach this threshold, it is very exhilarating. You may also feel a rushing of warmth or a flowing feeling that naturally occurs internally, throughout the body, as you release the breath and drift into relaxation.

If you feel a sense of frustration instead of satisfaction, it means that your body wishes it could get a more complete, full breath. It is actually quite typical for individuals who have not been using their full capacity to breathe deeply to experience this sense of frustration. Don't lose heart. Usually with regular practice the frustrated sense of not being able to gather a full breath will give way to a sense of satisfaction that feels like a big "Yes." One regular participant of the Wednesday Practice Session gave an inspiring testimonial after a period of regular practice: "I finally got a full breath," she said. "What a glorious feeling!"

With the inhalation, feel your rib cage and diaphragm expanding. On the exhalation, consciously allow yourself to relax deeply. Within two to three of these slow, deep breaths, you may begin to perceive an actual sensation: the healer within. Frequently this will feel like a spreading warmth that is most obvious in your hands, through your chest area, or in your cheeks. This is the sensation of your own body producing and circulating powerful self-healing resources, profound internal medicines.

Application Suggestions

○ *Health maintenance:* Do ten of these in a session set aside for this purpose; this takes just three minutes. Only very rarely has anyone complained of hyperventilation (feeling faint). Any time someone does repeated deep breathing dizziness may occur briefly. Just discontinue the practice, use fewer repetitions the next time, and then build up the number gradually. Or do the Essential Breath as often as you can remember; see the Remembering Breath, which follows.

○ *Health improvement:* Do ten repetitions two to three times a day, a total of ten minutes or less.

○ *Disease intervention:* Refer to the Remembering Breath. Use the Essential Breath continuously throughout the day.

○ *Getting started:* Begin by setting aside some health enhancement time each day in which you include a set of Essential Breaths. Or, try ten Essential Breaths as you fall asleep and ten when you wake, before you rise. Any time you remember to do this simple breath throughout the day you have done yourself a favor.

Benefits

The breath pumps the lymph as the diaphragm compresses the abdominal organs and the pressure in the chest cavity compresses the large lymph duct in the chest. In addition, you have to relax in order to take a deep breath, unless you are in the midst of strenuous exercise. The relaxation that accompanies a deep breath reduces constriction of the blood vessels and reduces blood pressure. The deep breath itself does not enhance oxygen delivery. The relaxation, however, does expand the capillaries so healing blood can penetrate deeper into the system. Relaxed breathing is accompanied by a shift in the production of brain chemicals and a shift into a slower brain-wave frequency, usually "alpha." Both foster natural healing activity.

The Remembering Breath

This technique brings the consciousness of the breath and the benefits of breath practice to as many of your daily activities as possible. In place of the concentrated effect of doing breathing exercises for a specific period of time, this method spreads the benefits of breath practice throughout the day.

The Remembering Breath is the same as the Essential Breath except that it is done every time you can remember to do it. Fill both the upper and lower parts of the lungs completely. As you exhale, allow yourself to relax deeply for a moment. Then go on with your normal activities, breathing as usual. After a while, initiate another deep, full breath. Notice that when you take a really full breath, you must adjust your posture and shift your attention. The posture shift, the attention shift, and the breath itself combine to become a dramatic self-healing tool.

The system for remembering is best established by each individual. The point is not so much to count the number of Essential Breaths you take as it is to become conscious of the breath and to initiate numerous deep Remembering Breaths throughout the day. It could as easily be ten or twelve full breaths per hour, or a deep breath every five minutes, every fifteen minutes, every ten or twenty breaths, every time you think of chocolate or smoking a cigarette, or every time the phone rings.

Because you must be conscious enough to decide or to remember to breathe deeply in this way, the Remembering Breath is actually a consciousness tool. In every tradition for spiritual enlightenment or consciousness enhancement, the breath is typically used as the starting place for the practice of meditation, prayer, and the pursuit of enlightened being.

Patients (health seekers) and workshop participants who have digital watches have set their alarms to remind them to take this breath. Another technique is to place colored sticker dots (available at office supply stores) on phones, mirrors, doors, and so on as constant reminders. We have developed a small reminder device with a quiet, soothing chime that can be set to remind you to do this practice (see page 257 for resources). Every time you see a colored sticker or hear a chime, you are reminded: "Oh, yes, the Remembering Breath." A lot of advantages are rolled into one with this breathing method: it can be used any time, it triggers positive physiological activities, it enhances consciousness, and it can be linked to stress mastery and the pursuit of inner peace throughout the day.

The Remembering Breath can also be linked to the process of giving life to a new behavior pattern. It can be used to help stop smoking, stop negative internal dialogue, or start a new habit by adding brief affirmations. When the desire to smoke arises, breathe deeply and affirm, "I love the feeling of a deep breath more than anything I experience from smoking." When negative inner talk is haunting you, take a deep breath and declare, "With this breath I expel the fear that this chatter within me expresses," and replace it with the voice of self-respect, which says "I can accomplish whatever I focus my creativity on." Or, "This breath neutralizes anxiety and nourishes tranquillity."

The Remembering Breath can be used to remember someone in prayer or to affirm a certain situation. It can be used to celebrate or honor the remembrance of something or someone precious, cherished, or beloved. With the Remembering Breath I frequently affirm my gratitude for inspiring work, healthy children, or the blessing of grace and creativity in my marriage. Often I use the moment of the Remembering Breath to send a prayer or deliver light to someone in my family, to one of my patients or students, or to one of the world's leaders.

Every time you remember to take a deep breath, take a moment on the exhalation to focus on a purposeful, positive thought, such as "I am an expression of God's creativity" or "I

am moved forward by universal wisdom." This can help to neutralize negative thoughts that may be hindering your potential.

It has been evident at the Health Action Clinic that those
people who become conscious enough to allow new health practices into their lives frequently have clinical results that medical
science would label dramatic. The Remembering Breath is a truly
extraordinary practice. When you master it, you will literally be a
new person. Nothing but the habitual inability to remember or
the compulsive addiction to complexity, busyness, or negative
inner dialogue would keep someone who is in need of healing
from doing this practice constantly throughout the day. This
method is truly the profound within the simple.

Application Suggestions

o *Health maintenance:* As often as you like or as often as you can
   remember to breathe deeply. Link it to redesigning yourself in
   the image that you wish to become.
o *Health improvement:* Remember to breathe deeply more often.
   Establish a system of remembrance triggers to remind you to initiate the breath frequently.
o *Disease intervention:* This breath practice is a powerful healer.
   Sincerely turn your awareness, attention, and intention to this
   practice, and you will experience dramatic benefits. Create a
   plan for remaining conscious enough to embrace the benefits of
   this powerful practice. Start with a few repetitions. Build up to a
   Remembering Breath every ten to twenty minutes.

Benefits

The deep breath pumps the lymph. The relaxation associated
with releasing a deep breath shifts the function of the autonomic
nervous system toward homeostasis. The capillary circulation
tends to be more open when you sustain a relaxed state. Oxygen-
and nutrition-bearing blood is able to penetrate more effectively
toward the tissues that need healing. It shifts the neurotransmitter profile toward natural restoration activities and slows the
brain-wave frequency toward the alpha, or self-healing, range.

The benefit of each individual deep breath may be small, but
if you remember to do this activity thirty to seventy times a day,

the accumulated benefit is dramatic. Doing the Remembering Breath every ten minutes over sixteen waking hours gives you a total of ninety-six deep breaths in a day. This generates a radical dose of the naturally occurring medicine within.

A Sigh of Relief

A Sigh of Relief is one the most powerful self-healing tools that we have. Unfortunately, most people do not use it until they are frustrated and angry. As a general rule it is preferable to release rather than store anger, frustration, anxiety, and worry. Science has proven that these emotions actually sabotage the immune system and other self-healing mechanisms by producing poisonous chemicals within the body. Physicians Walter Cannon (1945), and, later, Hans Selye (1978) suggested this body-mind connection early on, and a flood of research has continued to confirm it since. Better to use the Sigh of Relief to release tension before it produces such negative effects.

The Sigh of Relief can be combined with the Spontaneous Movement practice (page 51) to create a phenomenal self-healing method. It can also be used with the Front and Back Bending of the Spine (page 44). The Sigh of Relief complements any of the self-massage methods. When you find areas of soreness, use the Sigh of Relief to optimize the medicine within.

Breathe in, as in the Essential Breath, using the diaphragm. On the exhalation release an audible sigh. The sigh can be a sweet, relaxed, soft sigh expressing restfulness and trust; visualize peace and safety. Or it can be a loud groan, freeing accumulated frustration, anxiety, and other tensions; visualize traffic jams, the boss, too much work. Do this several times. Pay close attention to the sensations you experience. The Sigh of Relief gets your internal medicine moving immediately. You can actually feel it.

When I lectured on self-healing and health enhancement methods for the Wellness Committee at the American Medical Association (AMA) meeting in Chicago, the Sighs of Relief elicited from the audience were somewhat repressed. It took a while for the participants to loosen up and get out some good sighs. While at the Annual Wellness Conference at the University of Wisconsin, on the other hand, the participants let loose with robust relief-producing sighs with little coaching. Halfhearted or repressed Sighs of Relief have a limited effect because the person is too tense to allow the tool to do its work. Let your sighs be deep expressions that give you a genuine sense of relief.

Application Suggestions

- *Health maintenance:* As soon as you feel tension building up in your system. Use this practice as prevention.
- *Health improvement:* Use the method more often. Find a way to be more aware of when tension is just beginning to build up. Sigh for relief often.
- *Disease intervention:* This practice is a powerful healing too. Use it often. Even if you are limited in your movement or must spend time in bed, it dramatically activates the healer within.
- *Getting started:* Create a system for being aware of inner tension. Notice that small sighs as prevention are just as good as large ones when things have gotten out of hand.

Benefits

- Deep breaths are the best lymph pump. The relaxation on the sigh shifts the function of the autonomic nervous system and releases healing neurotransmitters into the system. The capillary circulation opens up when tension is released, which dramatically reduces blood pressure and the risk of heart attack.

  Research has found that up to 75 percent of doctor visits are for health problems that are complicated by stress and tension. The Sigh of Relief alone could cut medical visits significantly.

In, In, Out: Two Inhalations, One Exhalation

Our habitual tendency is to be lazy with our breathing. A breath practice that is easy to learn and apply and that has profound benefits is the "In, In, Out" method. You simply inhale twice, followed by a single exhalation to empty everything. The same pattern is repeated.

There are numerous variations on this method. Allow the first inhalation to be an abdominal breath that fills the lower lobes of the lungs and expands the lower belly area. Allow the second inhalation to fill the upper lobes of the lungs and expand the rib cage. Follow with one single exhalation. Or just use two deep inhalations that are full and slow and deep with complete filling of the lungs, followed by one complete exhalation to empty the lungs.

In one more variation the breaths are less full but sharper; they are quicker and more intense but take in less volume. Over a series of these breaths, more air is inspired on the double inhalations and less is expired on the exhalation. Over a series of ten to fifteen breath cycles, this creates a greater filling of the lungs and less emptying. Overall, on completion of this variation you could say that you are "fully inspired." The state of inspiration fosters positive thinking and positive action. Inspiration triggers the healing biochemistry of the medicine within.

You may add some movement of the hands when you use this method. On the inhalation lift the hands, palms up, from the navel to about the solar plexus or the heart in a gentle lifting movement, coordinated with the breathing. Then turn the palms down, and press slowly downward on the exhalation to about the level of the navel.

Or just walk and use In, In, Out breathing as you go. My mother actually taught me this walking and breathing practice early in my medical career after she had learned it in a workshop. And long before I began my work as a doctor of Chinese medicine, my high school track coach taught me to do the In, In, Out breathing to increase endurance in long-distance running.

Another variation on this method is widely used in China. Millions of cancer patients have used the unique Qigong (Chi Kung) method suggested by the Cancer Recovery Society. This simple method combines a walking form of Qigong with In, In, Out breathing. In Chinese the word for breathing in is *xi,* pronounced "she." The word for breathing out is *hu,* pronounced "who." So this practice is called *xi, xi, hu* ("she, she, who").

The cancer patient does the "in, in, out" pattern in conjunction with a slow, stylized walking in a state of deep relaxation or meditation. Members of the Cancer Recovery Society are either currently recovering from cancer or have recovered but continue with the practice as a form of prevention. Several of the members were diagnosed with cancer up to thirty years ago and feel that this walking form of self-healing has been the key to their long-term survival and health.

When a person is severely ill and unable to walk or when the person is near death, recovered members of the society will simply teach them *xi, xi, hu*. They tell inspiring stories of the thousands of surviving members of the society who have used this self-healing method to pull themselves back from the brink of death. In such cases the person is encouraged and supported by the society members to repeat the *xi, xi, hu* exercise as often as possible without becoming fatigued. After a time these patients are able to add some gentle movement to the breathing, even while lying in a hospital bed. When they have regained their strength enough to sit in the chair, they do *xi, xi, hu* sitting. When they can stand, they do it standing. Eventually, they combine the breathing with the walking technique.

On the inhalation feel the tendency of the body to lift upright. Do not lift the shoulders, however; instead, lead with the top of the head upward. Allow the filling of your lungs and rib cage to adjust your posture. Allow your head to float upward so that it sits gently atop your upright spine. Feel the difference between this posture and the way you usually sit or stand (see page 35).

Application Suggestions

- *Health maintenance:* Ten to fifteen repetitions, one session per day.
- *Health improvement:* Ten to thirty repetitions in two or more sessions per day.
- *Disease intervention:* Start *slowly* and build up to fifteen or more repetitions in several sessions per day.
- *Getting started:* Two to three repetitions, once or twice per day. Remember to build up slowly; more is better only when it is contributing to your health.

Benefits

Any deep breathing method pumps the lymphatic fluids. This one particularly accelerates the lymph in the chest cavity by radically increasing the pressure inside the rib cage. Because the inhalation is so full, the diaphragm presses down on the abdominal organs, which include several major lymph vessels and cavities. The rib cage expands and maintains its flexibility, and the tremendous pressure in the rib cage drives the thoracic vertebrae subtly upward, allowing the disks between the vertebae to fluff up like little pillows.

The members of the Chinese Cancer Recovery Society feel that this breath practice has saved many lives. When it is added to the gentle walking exercises, they believe it is an even more powerful healing tool. They feel very strongly that while there are authentic physiological benefits to the practice, the most important effect is to enhance and mobilize the internal healing energy called Qi (Chi).

The Gathering Breath

Sitting down, with the hands starting in the lap, or standing in the Preliminary Posture with the hands dangling at the sides begin to inhale and move the hands outward and upward as if you are scooping something useful, even precious, from the air around

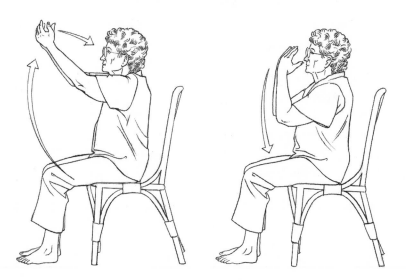

you. When your hands are slightly above and in front of you, the inhalation should be complete. Then bring your hands, side by side, palms facing you, toward your head. Then move them slowly down in front of your face, in front of your chest, in front of your abdomen, exhaling. When your hands reach the navel area, linger for a moment and then repeat.

Many people find this breath practice very calming. It is a kind of meditation that allows for some gentle movement, which often makes it easier for people to relax. Frequently, people who have a hard time meditating find it easier if some mild movement is involved. Many who have found it difficult to take a full, deep breath have discovered that the arm movement helps to open up the rib cage and fill the lungs. Allow yourself to relax deeply during this practice.

In China this movement and breath practice is part of a powerful Qigong method called "marrow washing," which gathers energy (Qi) from nature and then purposefully stores it in the marrow of the bones, like electrical potential in a battery. As the hands pass over the body, focus intently on the energy penetrating through the surface of the body, through the flesh and muscles, and through the surface of the bones to be stored in the marrow. This stored energy becomes an available resource to vitalize the organs and glands, harmonize imbalances, and heal disease. Allow yourself to float free of concerns and simplify your thoughts. Move toward a state of mental neutrality where you are simultaneously cheerful and indifferent.

You may, if you wish, imagine or visualize that you are gathering healing energy from around you—from the universe, heaven, God, or a marvelous pool of healing waters. Bathe yourself gently in this rich resource. Allow the healing energy to penetrate deeply in order to nourish the organs and glands.

You may want to turn and face the different directions. From the east gather the energy of spring, of awakening and sprouting. From the south gather the energy of summer, of maturing and ripening. From the west gather the energy of autumn, the reward of the harvest. From the north gather the energy of winter, of patience and rest.

As you relax in this practice you may feel the warmth of your hands as they pass in front of your face. The Chinese call this "Qi sensation." Rest in the rhythm of the movement, allowing the breath to be natural as you go deeper into relaxation. Notice that very soon you begin to feel carefree, lighter. You may become aware of a soothing floating sensation that makes you feel filled with lightness, as if the cells are less compressed, less dense.

Application Suggestions

- *Health maintenance:* Five to ten repetitions in one session per day.
- *Health improvement:* Ten to fifteen repetitions, or add a second practice session.
- *Disease intervention:* Start slowly and build up to fifteen to twenty repetitions.
- *Getting started:* Two to three repetitions, once or twice a day. This method is very mild, so feel free to do as many as you like.

Benefits

The movement of the arms increases the lymph flow in the chest and shoulder area, which makes this practice particularly helpful in preventing or resolving disorders and discomforts in the chest and neck area. Be sure to combine significant expansion of the upper ribs with the lifting of the arms. The rib cage is expanded and lung capacity is increased. The deep inhalation causes the diaphragm to compress the abdominal organs, which triggers the elimination of metabolic by-products from the intracellular spaces—spaces between the cells in the organs and glands.

Because the intention of this practice is to calm the mind and deepen your relaxation, it has a strong effect on your neurochemistry, enhancing the naturally occurring internal mechanisms that support self-healing and self-restoration through the autonomic nervous system and the immune system.

Remember, if you find it interesting, to be aware of the circulation of the energy that the Chinese refer to as the Qi. It is astonishing that the ancient Chinese, with no scientific knowledge of the actual physiology of the bone marrow or of its value, had an intuitive sense that the marrow was where vitality is stored. All red and white blood cells and almost all immune cells are born in the marrow. Somehow the Chinese intuition was quite enlightened regarding self-healing thousands of years ago.

CHAPTER 7

Method 4

Deep Relaxation and Meditation Practices

A quiet mind cureth all.

Robert Burton,
English clergyman, author,
1577–1640

WHEN AN INDIVIDUAL PURPOSEFULLY SEEKS A STATE OF deep relaxation, a number of important physiological mechanisms are triggered. The relaxed state, called the "relaxation response" by Dr. Herbert Benson of Harvard University, is the opposite of the "fight or flight" state, which has also been called the "stress response" (Benson, 1975, 1996). Researchers have found that many diseases are caused or aggravated by stress, which causes overactivity of the sympathetic nervous system and exhaustion of the adrenal glands. They have also found that inducing the relaxation response can resolve or neutralize the negative effects of stress on the body and heal disease.

In biofeedback—a highly researched method for reducing head and neck pain, high blood pressure, syndromes of gastrointestinal discomfort, and anxiety—the primary technique is to initiate and sustain a deeply relaxed state. Research has indicated that the physiological mechanisms that are triggered by inducing relaxation are

○ Reduction of blood pressure
○ Warming of the skin surface due to the dilation of blood capillaries
○ Enhanced productivity of healing neurochemicals and hormones
○ A shift toward a lower frequency of brain-wave activity (alpha and theta)

In deep relaxation, biofeedback, meditation practice, and the process of visualization, the induction of the relaxation response precedes and accompanies the successful initiation of each technique. Most of the great spiritual traditions of both the East and the West initiate the deeper levels of spiritual practice by eliciting the relaxation response. Dr. Benson himself, when in China to research some of the more fantastic aspects of Qigong (Chi Kung), stated that he felt the primary effect was triggered by an initial induction of the relaxation response. The Chinese call this the Qigong state. In ancient cultures, prayer, meditation, ritual, and contemplation were all initiated by shifting into the relaxed state.

For self-healing and health enhancement there are many simple yet highly effective techniques for achieving deep relaxation. Deeper or altered states of consciousness may also be attained by merely remaining mindful of the breath alone. In such methods the individual refines his or her practice to the extent that the busy mind is completely quieted or emptied. This is less easy to accomplish than simple relaxation. Average, busy-minded people benefit from starting with some preliminary methods of relaxation because these are easier to learn and apply. They allow you to focus your mind rather than trying to empty or quiet it completely. Success with these simple relaxation practices may lead, over time, to an interest in more advanced practices.

In the ancient Asian traditions of health care and medicine, the goal of the various approaches to self-applied health enhancement is to gather, refine, and circulate life force or bio-energy, the Qi (Chi). In the gentle movement, self-massage, and breath practices that we have learned and in the following relaxation practices, one confirmation of success is to feel the sensation of internal resources circulating. It is very common to experience sensations of heat or tingling in the hands. This energy may also be sensed as a flowing, pouring, or circulating feeling or as a sensation of puffiness.

The hands are one of the most sensitive organs of the human body. You can presume that when you feel the sensation in your hands, the same activity is present in organs that are less sensitive, like the liver, the kidneys, and even the glands. If you do not feel this sensation, don't worry; the benefits are still occurring. It often takes some months or even longer to begin to have these perceptions. Once you have begun to feel this sensation in the hands, it will be easier to recognize in other parts of the body, such as the feet, the cheeks, or the abdomen around the belly button.

An entire science, psychoneuroimmunology (PNI), is based on the idea that our state of mind (psyche) initiates activities through the nervous system that have an effect on the immune system. The single most transformative scientific finding that confirmed the presence of the healer within for the Western mind was when Dr. Candace Pert and her team at the National Institutes for Health (NIH) found that the body produces its own pain medication internally (Pert 1985, 1997). These chemicals, called neurotransmitters or "information substances," are literally the biochemistry of thoughts and feelings. This validated the ancient Chinese idea, originally perceived as a poetic metaphor, that we actually produce a healing elixir within.

The psyche includes the emotional, attitudinal, and intellectual components of oneself. Knowledge, choice, and feeling are all aspects of the psyche. Through knowledge and choice one may elect to trigger the benefits of contemplation and affirmation. Take a deep breath, relax, and repeat internally, "My body, mind, and spirit are always working to keep me supremely well."

If a person has internally agreed to make choices that equate with joy, satisfaction, and trust, then a positive physiological response occurs throughout the body, particularly in the immune system. In the past this was called positive thinking or mental healing. We will discuss more of these attitudinal aspects of self-healing in chapter 11.

The "psychoneuro" aspect of psychoneuroimmunology can be linked with other systems besides the immune system. Psychoneurocardiology is the use of the mind to initiate activities in the body, mind, and spirit that have an impact on the heart and circulatory system. Psychoneuroendocrinology affects the endocrine glands. The endocrine glands produce hormones that include the powerful chemicals used by the body for healing. Psychoneurogastroenterology reflects the effect of mind and emotions on the digestive system.

One of my patients was a firefighter. His case demonstrates the benefit of meditation and the direct connection between the psyche and the organs. He experienced "acid reflux," a disorder in which strong stomach acid wells up and damages the tissue of the esophagus (throat). He reported experiencing a painful burning sensation almost every day.

The acid often burns and causes scar tissue in the passageway to the stomach. Several times his doctor had to expand the damaged tissue by performing a procedure called "endoscopic dilatation," in which a large carrot-shaped device is lowered deep into the throat and suddenly springs open—a painful and frightening experience. Finally, at a recent visit, the doctor had diagnosed tissue changes indicating cancer of the esophagus.

The firefighter came for acupuncture feeling desperate. I asked if his physician had instructed him in meditation. "No," he said. He threw himself into meditation earnestly every day. The burning sensation ceased within the first week.

A couple of months later he returned for a follow-up. He was very positive. The doctor suggested that urgency for cancer treatment had diminished since the "reflux" had reduced. The burning had been a problem only once, during a period of extra stress. He felt angry that his physician had not known the value of meditation, but he was visibly relieved to have gained such a powerful self-healing tool that eliminated the need for what he called the "exploding carrot."

Most experts in the field of mind-body medicine and healing agree that both meditation and prayer are forms of focused intention. Both produce relaxation and shifts in brain-wave frequency and body chemistry. Edgar Cayce (1877–1945), an American mystic who advocated holistic thinking when conventional medicine had almost forgotten about natural healing and the medicine within, stated, "In prayer we talk with God, in meditation we listen." The role of prayer in healing has gotten attention in research (Byrd, 1988) and has helped kindle national interest in the religious community regarding church-based health programming. The rapidly growing Health Ministries Association fosters health care in churches, including parish nursing and healing prayer.

In the Chinese tradition, where energy pathways and acupuncture points are accepted aspects of the body, attention during relaxation practices is directed to specific points and energy channels. In India the chakras, or energy centers, related to the endocrine organs and nerve centers (plexuses) are the focus of attention as the practitioner goes deeper and deeper into a state of relaxation. Relaxation, meditation, contemplation, and prayer are thought to maximize the flow of vital energies called Qi and Prana.

The following relaxation practices are powerful yet simple tools that you can use to complement medical treatment, accelerate self-healing, or optimize your performance, productivity, and endurance in either work or play. Integrating these practices with gentle movement, self-massage, and breathing practices heightens their effectiveness. Of the four essential self-healing methods, relaxation is really the central, most primary one. It complements and strengthens the others.

Progressive Relaxation

Mentally bring your awareness to each part of your body progressively and then consciously relax that part, from the feet all the way up to your head. Your breath should be full and relaxed. Notice that this process takes only five minutes. It is particularly easy to do in bed before sleep, on awakening, or in the hospital. It can even be adapted for use at work.

o In a comfortable position (lying, sitting, or you may even adapt for standing), close your eyes and take ten slow deep breaths.
o Bring your awareness to your right leg. Inhale deeply and lift the leg up slightly, tensing the foot and leg. Tense them tighter. Then exhale and let the leg drop gently. Roll the leg from side to side and relax. Inhale and repeat the same for the left leg and foot.
o Now bring your attention to your thighs and buttocks. Inhale, and contract your buttocks, pelvic muscles, and thighs. Tighten until the end of the breath and then release and exhale.
o Now bring your attention to your right arm. Inhale, raise, and tense your right arm, making your hand into a fist. Tense and

hold. Exhale and drop the arm gently. Roll the right arm from side to side. Inhale and repeat with the left arm.

○ Inhale and bring the shoulder blades together in back. Squeeze tightly, then release, exhaling.
○ Inhale and bring both shoulders up to your ears. Hold them up. Then, exhale and let them down. Repeat three times.
○ Inhale and tighten the facial muscles. Make your face into a prune, squeezing tightly. Exhale and release the tension.
○ Roll your head gently from side to side.
○ Continue, with a few more relaxed breaths, to go deeper and deeper into relaxation.

This technique is perfect for those who wish to tap the benefits of the relaxation methods but have little prior experience. In every tradition where health-enhancing techniques have been refined over thousands of years, the distracted mind is considered one of the great challenges to the practice. Even the great meditation masters call their daily system of quieting the mind a "practice." It is not a finished product but an ongoing "practice." Even the experts are constantly refining their ability to quiet the mind in order to benefit the body.

This particular technique ensures a genuine state of relaxation by actually involving the body parts. In most meditation techniques it is possible for the thoughts to wander. Just the mind is involved, and it is difficult to be consciously free of thought. In this relaxation method it is quickly obvious when your mind has wandered because you will stop the contracting and releasing of the body parts. Only three things could possibly have occurred. Either you consciously elected to discontinue ("I think I'll stop this process"), or you have become distracted by your wandering mind, or you have fallen asleep.

When the mind drifts, the process stops. When you realize you are no longer engaged in the process, say to yourself, "This is a practice that I am perfecting. I forgive myself for forgetting and congratulate myself for remembering to return to the process." Then simply continue.

If you have drifted into sleep, it is especially important to understand the healing effect of rest. Frequently, people have the attitude that needing rest means laziness. Balance in life means that action and rest are in harmony. It is not unusual for people to work or play hard but then neglect rest. If you fall asleep during meditation, call it creative napping, and celebrate that you are getting some needed rest. One of the most frequent prescriptions I have made as a doctor includes sleep, napping, and vacation. Eventually, your need for rest will be fulfilled, and it will become easier to meditate.

Take a moment to be aware of the results of this practice. You will feel refreshed and rested. If it leaves you sleepy, please understand that you probably need rest. If you are alert, you can actually feel the physiological sensation of the healer within.

Variation

A variation on this progressive relaxation uses visualization, affirmation, and inner dialogue. Remember the guidelines: vary your practice of the methods, keep your practice easy, and tailor your practice to be fun. Feel free to adapt your practice so that it works for you.

This method can be done sitting or lying down, and it can be done as a standing meditation. Allow the breath to be full and relaxed, not urgent. Deeply relax and visualize each of the body parts relaxing or filling up with healing energies. Visualize the parts that you are addressing glowing radiantly with vitality. On each inhalation bring your attention to the next area of the body. On the exhalation relax the area and silently affirm the following to yourself:

1 Now my feet and toes are relaxed.
2 Now my calves up to my knees are deeply relaxed.
3 Now my thighs are completely relaxed.
4 Now my buttocks are completely relaxed.
5 Now my hands and fingers are completely relaxed.
6 Now my arms are fully relaxed.
7 Now the muscles and organs in my pelvis are relaxed.
8 Now the muscles and organs in my abdomen are deeply relaxed.
9 Now my chest is completely relaxed.
10 Now my back is relaxed.
11 Now my shoulders are relaxed.
12 Now my neck is fully relaxed.

13 Now my face and jaw are relaxed.
14 Now my eyes are deeply relaxed.
15 Now my temples and forehead are relaxed.
16 Now my scalp is relaxed.
17 Now my head is totally relaxed.

Notice this takes just seventeen deep breaths. Each breath lasts about ten seconds. Seventeen breaths times ten seconds equals 170 seconds, which is a little less than three minutes—not a great deal of time out of your day. This same practice can be done with many more awareness points, which may include focusing on each finger and toe, segments of the arms and legs, specific joints, individual organs, and so on (from thirty to seventy awareness points).

When you have relaxed through these seventeen areas and feel you could benefit from a deeper level of relaxation, go through the areas again. When you feel you have attained a significantly deep state of relaxation, turn your attention to inner healing. If the gastrointestinal system is a part of your health challenge, bring your awareness to that area of the body. Visualize the stomach and intestines operating optimally. Acknowledge that the stomach and the intestines are charged with all the life force that they need. See them, in your mind's eye, glowing radiantly with vitality and healing.

If one of your health challenges is cold hands, or if discomfort in your hands is more severe as in arthritis, Raynaud's disease, or scleroderma, then after the general relaxation, bring your awareness to your hands. Visualize or imagine that your hands are in the sun, resting beside you as you nap comfortably at the beach. Actually feel heat in your hands. In your mind's eye visualize the capillaries, which are very small blood vessels, becoming large tubes that carry larger volumes of warm blood from the center of the body into the hands. Patients at risk for stroke and with migraines have learned to control the blood flow to various parts of the body using this simple technique.

If your heart needs healing, then after the preliminary relaxation, bring your awareness to the heart, and visualize healing resources migrating there to nourish and support the heart's function. If headaches are your major discomfort, bring the focus to the head, and visualize fresh air filling your head, or imagine a cooling sensation dissipating excess tension. If it is clear to you that the head pain is caused by too much tension or blood flow in the upper body, then bring the awareness to the hands and feet and visualize the pain flowing out of the head. This will help to bring the energy down from the upper body to be released through the feet and the fingertips. Again, visualize the veins, arteries, and capillaries expanding to become large pipes, rather than tiny vessels. While the image of pipes carrying massive amounts of blood to the hands and feet may seem extreme, it is a powerful visualization that has helped many people with high blood pressure, headaches, shoulder and neck pain, ulcers, insomnia, and even more serious disorders like cancer and AIDS.

The ability to adjust internal function consciously, to slow the heart rate, warm the hands, reduce oxygen consumption, and so on are called "voluntary physiological controls." At the Menninger Institute, Alyce and Elmer Green, who did breakthrough work on biofeedback, found that voluntary physiological control could be learned by anyone and that the effects on health are dramatic (Green, 1977).

For a very brief but remarkable dose of the most profound medicine, use this same sequence to do a rapid full-body scan. Inhale slowly, and as you exhale scan the whole body, consciously relaxing and releasing any tension that you find. You can apply this while on hold on the telephone, sitting in the dentist's chair, riding in the subway, bus, or taxi, and even in a team meeting at work. It happens fast, no one knows but you, and the benefits over time are significant.

Application Suggestions

- *Health maintenance:* One session per day.
- *Health improvement:* One to two sessions per day.
- *Disease intervention:* Start slowly and build up to two or more sessions per day.
- *Getting started:* One brief session per day. Notice how easy this can be. Confirm the simple but extraordinary value of this practice by doing it vigilantly for a couple of weeks.

Gathering Nature's Healing Resources

In the relaxation and meditation traditions of the ancient cultures, the regulation of the mind goes beyond simply focusing on the body. In the Native American tradition, nature is the source of all life and healing. In the Christian tradition, contemplation is focused on divine grace and the light of spirit.

In both Qigong and Yoga, one purposefully draws healing energy and the light of spirit from nature and the universe. Rather than limiting your attention to specific body parts such as arms, legs, or organs, as in the previous practices, you visualize the function of internal resources (such as vitality or life force), passageways, and gateways. Traditional Chinese medicine holds that energy can be gathered from water, mountains, trees, and the universe through nearly a thousand acupuncture energy gates (points) distributed over the body's surface.

The energy of the heaven, called yang, is naturally drawn down toward the earth. The energy of the earth, called yin, is naturally drawn up toward heaven. These two rich universal resources are considered to be the essential energies of life and health as they circulate and interact in the world and in the human body. At the surface of the earth where these energies mix is the realm of biological life, the biosphere. The Chinese, as well as the Indians who live south of the Himalayan mountains, believe that one can draw intentionally on the energy of the heaven, the earth, and the biosphere to enhance and harmonize one's own personal energy.

Start by getting comfortable—either standing in the Preliminary Posture (page 35), sitting, or lying down. Allow your breath to be deep, slow, and relaxed.

With each inhalation you are gathering the resource of oxygen. At the same time imagine, visualize, or feel (if you can) that you are also gathering in vitality (Qi) from the heaven, the earth, and the biosphere through thousands of energy gateways. The Chinese believe that this absorption of energy is always in process in order to sustain life. However, in this practice you are increasing the extent to which it is occurring because you have focused your attention and intention on self-healing. Ancient cultures and religious traditions believe that the life energies react to our thoughts and intentions. Current research from numerous disciplines, particularly on neurotransmitters or "information substances," suggests that this is true.

On your exhalations, allow yourself to slip deeper and deeper into relaxation. Visualize the internal healing resources circulating throughout the system in the energy channels. Recall Tracing the Acupuncture Energy Channels (page 70)—the life energy flows up the front and down the back. You may feel waves of warmth, tingling, or a flowing feeling. It is not necessary to know the channel pathways specifically. This all happens automatically. Just celebrate the flow of vitality throughout your system. Visualize it going to the organs. You can place your hands on the liver, spleen, kidneys, heart, and umbilical area as described in chapter 5 under "Energizing the Organs" (page 74). You may feel energy or warmth passing from your hands into the organs.

On your inhalations, you are gathering healing resources. On your exhalations, affirm the power of those resources circulating within to increase health and vitality. Focus your attention carefully inside, and you may actually feel the internal medicine working.

Continue this practice for five to fifteen minutes. Inhale, gathering healing resources through breath and through the thousands of acupuncture gates. On the exhalation, focus on the circulation of healing resources internally. Over the period of your practice you will feel deeply relaxed. Use your mind's intention to direct the flow of the internal healing forces to the organs or body parts that need healing the most.

Application Suggestions

- *Health maintenance:* One session per day.
- *Health improvement:* One or two sessions per day.
- *Disease intervention:* Start slowly and build up to two or more brief sessions per day.
- *Getting started:* Begin to build an awareness of the richness of nature's healing potential by beginning with a brief session—five to seven minutes—of this practice.

Mindfulness and Insight

This practice, called mindfulness or insight meditation, is really simple to describe. There is only one focus; in other words, you want to sustain a single point of awareness. This focus is usually the sensation of the breath as it passes into and out of the nose. Stand, sit, or lie down comfortably and begin to notice the breath. There is a cool sensation as fresh air enters the nose and a warm sensation as the exhalation exits from the nose. When your mind is attracted to a passing thought, simply return your focus to the breath.

The goal of this practice is to free the body from the effects of the busy mind. When a thought takes your attention from the single point of focus, you may still be quiet and somewhat relaxed, but the body is affected by the busyness of mind. When you are able to sustain awareness of the breath, only just for a few moments, the body is freed completely from the effect of mind busyness. The healer within turns to the activity of producing its potent medicines.

It is beneficial for the body simply to stop *doing,* even if the mind has some involvement. In both previous methods—Progressive Relaxation and Gathering Nature's Resources—one stops, relaxes, and purposefully shifts the focus to relaxing certain body parts or gathering and directing healing resources. The mindfulness method, however, is particularly effective because you suspend all but one focus. You will discover that the mind is easily pulled into the thought stream. If nothing else, this practice will teach you how really busy your mind is. With compassion and forgiveness for yourself, patiently return to the sensation of the breath. Over time you will gain greater and greater skill in dismissing thoughts for a few moments a day.

Variations

There are several variations on the process of sustaining a single focus. When you enter the relaxed state with the eyes closed, there are two sensations that you may become aware of. Visually, you may become aware of light or color. Or you may become conscious of a whispering sound. Either one of these can become a single focus for meditation. There are elaborate traditions of light and sound meditation, but in the context of mindfulness and insight, the process can be stated quite simply.

Turn your attention to the light or color that appears in your visual awareness. Simply note it, celebrate it, enjoy it. When thought enters, notice that the light disperses or arranges into thought images. Notice that when you return to the light, the thought disperses. Attending to the thought and attending to the light are mutually exclusive; it is impossible to do both. Notice that the light brightens when you shift your attention from the eyes themselves, as the source of seeing, back to the place in your brain where sight actually occurs.

Similarly, to use the whisper within as your focus, first find the sound. It is usually a subtle hum or a whoosh or a high frequency whisper. Attend to the sound only, and all thoughts will disappear. In many traditions this sound is thought to be our link to the essential vibratory nature of the universe. In practical terms it is the sound of your life process—the flow of fluids, the transmission of nerve impulses, and the biological interactions within. Notice that when busyness of mind sets in, the sound disappears. When you return to the sound, the thoughts disappear.

Each of these points of focus—breath, sound, or light—is a means of awakening the healer within. Mindfulness and insight are not just powerful healing tools; they will also lead you to self-discovery and personal insight. When it is very difficult to suspend thought for a few moments, this is a powerful teaching. Obviously, thought is a powerful tool, one that has figured prominently in the evolution of human possibilities. How evolved is it, however, when one has a tool that one cannot elect to shut off?

Application Suggestions

- *Health maintenance:* One session per day.
- *Health improvement:* One or two sessions per day.
- *Disease intervention:* Start slowly and build up to two or more brief sessions per day.
- *Getting started:* Begin by occasionally shifting to the mindfulness and insight method when you are doing any meditation or relaxation practice. It is enlightening to check your ability to stay on a single focus.

Benefits

Relaxation triggers dozens of positive physiological mechanisms. The neurotransmitters, information molecules that are produced during deep relaxation, are powerful components of the medicine that we produce within us. Relaxation reduces pressure within the circulatory system by expanding the size of the capillaries, which prevents stroke, relieves heart pain, and reduces the risk of circulatory problems. This increases the surface area of the blood vessels, allowing for more effective delivery of blood, rich in oxygen and nutrition, into the tissues, organs, and glands.

The immune system, which is sabotaged by stress and tension, is supercharged by deep relaxation, because the relaxed state releases information molecules that attach to the immune cells and tell them how to operate. All diseases—cancer, heart disease, metabolic disease, obesity, anxiety, depression—are improved with relaxation practice. All the self-healing methods—movement, massage, breathing—are enhanced by relaxation.

Because we are generally addicted to complexity and busyness, reaching a state of authentic relaxation is a challenge. Many of us are locked into worry, hurry, overwork, and compulsive behaviors, and the mind is very difficult to quiet. The beauty of these particular methods is their simplicity. They allow the mind to have a focus. When the attention wanders off the process, just gently return your focus to the practice.

Be patient. It is useless to become stressed about your skill in meditation. Relax; rest in knowing that each time you engage in one of these practices you have done yourself a tremendous favor. Our goal for now is not enlightenment. Rather, we seek healing, vitality enhancement, and personal effectiveness. The quest for enlightenment is always an option, and these methods help to build a foundation for spiritual practice.

It is not far from deep relaxation and meditation to prayer. Quite a bit of research has demonstrated that the relaxed, focused intention that we call prayer has significant effects, which we will explore in chapter 13. With just a little effort you may shift from meditation into a state of prayerfulness during your practice time.

Part 3

THE PRACTICE

An ounce of prevention is better than a pound
of cure.
And a stitch in time saves nine.

Grandma

○

A profound and inspiring idea is only so
much fantasy until the beholder of the idea
takes action. In the case of health enhancement and self-healing, very small actions produce major results. This is like getting a whole
pound of cure for the cost of a single ounce of
prevention.

CHAPTER 8

Bringing the Methods into Your Life

He who has begun
has half done.
Dare to be wise—
Begin!

Horace,
ancient philosopher, 65–8 B.C.E.

AS YOU BEGIN TO USE THESE TOOLS YOU WILL QUICKLY face a number of challenging questions. Which practices should I do? How many? When in my busy day? Who can guide me in this? From over twenty years of experience with this body of information I know that the best answers to all of these questions will eventually come from you.

The next chapters intend to give you some guidance and inspiration as well as permission to develop and perfect your own personal approach to health enhancement and self-healing. At first you may think it is impossible to improve your own health by yourself without expert guidance. You are probably asking, "How could I know how to create and sustain a self-healing or personal empowerment practice?" This is a frequent question. Fortunately, the answer is easy. There are many ways. All you need in order to begin is a little enthusiasm and the willingness to try a few of the methods.

You will soon realize, if you haven't already, that everyone's practice is very personal. The *only* genuine way to improve your practice is through personal insight and refinement. The *only* genuine way to improve your health is by yourself. While the medical system can assist you with its expertise in naming and managing disease, actually enhancing health will be up to you. The history of medicine is a chain of events, from the bubonic plague to tuberculosis to cancer to AIDS, that has disease as a focus. Health, health maintenance, and health enhancement have only recently become focal points in the health care system.

To make this process of health enhancement and self-healing effective, fun, doable, and interesting, we each will eventually have to be willing to celebrate our self-reliance. By noticing and honoring your own strengths, limits, and preferences, you will be able to design a potent practice for yourself. Eventually, you will become an expert at modifying and adapting your practice. Rather than necessarily needing to find an expert or master teacher, you may become one for yourself.

Robert's Story

Robert's story demonstrates one person's answer to some of the questions you are asking. Robert, a retired engineer, did not allow the questions to stand in his way. He is more of a student than a patient. He just started in and then refined the process on his own. This is how he got started on the self-healing path, in his own words.

> After my retirement I decided to check on my health status with a routine physical. I have always been generally healthy, although I have experienced two kinds of headaches: tension headaches (I was a little surprised when these continued after my retirement) and sinus headaches. Otherwise, I have been quite well.
>
> The doctor reported that I was perfectly healthy and that he was impressed with all of my tests except for my blood pressure, which was somewhat elevated, and my PSA (prostate specific antigen), a test for prostate cancer, which was also slightly elevated. For the blood pressure he prescribed a medication. He showed concern for the prostate

reading, which was 4.3 (4 is the warning threshold), and recommended that we reevaluate in six months. I asked if there was anything preventive I could do. He answered that we would just have to wait and see.

Overall I felt good about being in better-than-average health for my age. However, I was haunted by the constant flow of information about prostate cancer and its high incidence that I was getting from the media. Over the years I had experienced an "ache" in the prostate area that grew worse with stress; now it became exaggerated. Several of my acquaintances had episodes with medications, surgical prostate removals, and radiation treatments. I was disturbed to see that they were simply not regaining their health and vitality, even with the help of renowned experts in the urology field.

Six months later I was horrified to have the PSA come back significantly elevated to a 9 (danger zone). I was immediately referred to a urologist, whose digital inspection revealed no dangerous signs, but I was not relieved. I then had a biopsy in which five out of six samples were clear. Only one was borderline. The physician felt that the risk was significant, however, and that we should begin planning the surgical removal of my prostate. He started to give me information as if I had already elected to proceed with the surgery.

I was really in a kind of shock. I kept asking if there was something I could do. Just as I was walking out the door, as an afterthought, the doctor mentioned that I might use my computer to check the Internet for on-line support groups for prostate patients. That evening I began a search of a number of Internet resources.

Right away the process helped me to decide to get a second opinion from another urologist. I was fascinated to find, as I was cruising here and there on the Internet, that in addition to radiation treatment there were many unusual alternatives for prostate cancer, including exercises, diets, herbal formulas, and treatments like acupuncture.

I began to print out information that quickly grew into a large file. I set up an appointment with a second urologist. I also set up appointments with two radiation specialists so I could get a first and second opinion on the radiation alternative as well. A third PSA test came back at 5, which produced little relief as the 9 now seemed like an anomaly, and if the 9 was a fluke reading, couldn't the 5 be a fluke as well?

By the time I had seen the second urology surgeon and the two radiation practitioners I was confused and angry. I was nervous that both urologists and now the radiologists were so ready to use invasive procedures based on a test that they all felt might be giving one or more false readings. It distressed me that the surgeons were urging only the surgery alternative and the radiation doctors were urging only the radiation alternative.

It became clear that they had little understanding or knowledge about which was better, or safer, or more effective. It began to seem instead like each was seeking my business. I found that none of them knew anything about the treatment alternatives that I had discovered on the Internet. And it seemed to have slipped everyone's mind that in my biopsy only one out of six specimens was on the borderline of showing cancer, digital evaluation showed no signs, and my PSA was currently only one point over the warning threshold of 4.

I began to hunt in the bookstore for more information on the self-healing methods and alternative therapies I had located on the Internet. I found a huge book called *Alternative Medicine: The Definitive Guide* that had an interesting section on prostate cancer. I was particularly drawn to the chapter on the self-healing practices of the Chinese called Qigong (Chi Kung) that included the practical physiological reasons why simple self-healing methods are beneficial. In addition it gave me a series of practices that I could begin to use right away. I was relieved to have something that I could do. I ordered an instructional video [see page 257] that helped to bring the self-healing practices alive for me. I became even more angry that not one of my doctors had recommended anything for me to do to help myself.

I began to use the self-healing methods described in the book and video. I also began to take the herb saw palmetto, which has been found in numerous studies to be a useful remedy for the prostate. After all of the confusion and frustration with the medical approach to my situation, I began to feel a lightening of my stress load. I felt empowered.

I was really amazed when very soon my headaches stopped. They have not returned in the several months of my practicing the self-healing methods. This was exciting confirmation to me that I was on a healing path. I called the physicians and told them I would not be having any procedures until I had worked with some personal healing for a while. I promised to have follow-up PSA tests to evaluate my level of risk, which seemed reasonable.

On the one hand, I felt it must be impossible that I could personally have such a powerful effect on my medical situation. On the other, I felt inspired by the same idea: I personally could have a beneficial effect on my case. A couple of times I thought I must need a teacher or somebody to tell me what to do or confirm that I was proceeding correctly. But then I began to realize that the improvement that I was experiencing was quite confirming in itself.

I just continued, trusting the concept that no matter what disease one is challenged with and no matter what therapeutic approach one is using to resolve the disease, one must remember to take vigilant personal action to enhance health as well. This is such a reasonable idea that I still wonder why my doctors were not trained to use this concept. I am so thankful to that doctor that suggested the Internet. That brief afterthought led to a chain of events that really changed everything.

I found myself enjoying the process of trying different things. Some of the practices seemed perfect for me and my lifestyle, others were less appealing. I was able to piece together a regimen of practices. I always felt—actually perceived—a sense of increased well-being every time I would use one or several of the methods. Over a period of weeks I was delighted to find that the ache in my prostate area diminished. Several prostate symptoms—frequent urination and discomfort—diminished as well.

This is not the best or most important part of Robert's story. When he finally came to the Health Action Clinic he was not saying, "I am sick, please get an expert to fix me." Instead he said, "I have been working with a serious health challenge. I would like your assistance in evaluating my health status from the perspective of Chinese medicine, and I would like your guidance on how I might improve my self-healing regimen." This is the attitude of an empowered, self-reliant individual.

The power of Robert's story isn't just in his discovery of self-healing and alternative thinking about medicine and disease. These are, of course, miracles in themselves. The spectacular lesson that Robert provides for us is that he grasped from the very beginning that he was allowed to take action to enhance his health himself. Probably due to some aspect of his upbringing or personality, Robert had not learned, as do most people, that he was not able (or allowed) to take such self-empowered actions.

Notice that he did not need a teacher, special knowledge, or certification to help himself. Nor did he need a doctor, although he did engage medical expertise to maintain a current diagnosis and track his progress. Somehow he understood it was his right and his responsibility to take action himself. He just experimented with this and that. Through personal trial and course correction, he refined a regimen of daily practices that was perfect for him.

This chapter is about how you, like Robert, can design your own set of practices. He wondered if he would do it wrong but worked his way through to a profound truth: no one else can do better in self-healing and health enhancement than a person can do for himself or herself.

Yes, we will call on physician expertise. Yes, it is critical to understand the medical or diagnostic situation. Yes, we will have facilitators, mentors, teachers, and guides. But it is not necessary to get permission to enhance your health from someone else. It is not necessary to be told what to do to heal yourself or what to do to enhance your medical treatment. These are things that each individual has the capacity and right to understand.

If you are willing to pay attention, then you are actually the best person to be the chief of staff on your case. Most physicians will celebrate your intuitive and innovative nature. Who can possibly know you better than you do? Who can possibly guide your personal improvement process better than you can?

Robert's Self-Healing Routine

When Robert eventually elected to visit the Health Action Clinic he wanted more than a Chinese medicine diagnosis, an acupuncture treatment, and herbal medicine. He stated clearly right away that his key goal for the visit was to review his self-healing plan and confirm his choices in the area of nutrition, herbs, and self-healing methods. It was not a surprise to find that his choice of practices was very well suited for his situation.

Robert began to explain his daily routine: "I've changed the routine around quite a bit; this is my current system. When I awaken in the morning, I do a series of deep breaths to get things going. I combine the deep breathing with Energize the Organs [page 74]. Then, sitting on the edge of the bed, I do massage of the hands, feet, and ears. I do the contracting and releasing exercise [Front and Back Bending of the Spine, page 44]. Then I stand and do tracing up the front and down the back [Tracing the Acupuncture Energy Channels, page 70] and the Spontaneous Movement [page 51]. Later I go on a forty- to forty-five-minute power walk with my wife.

"Throughout the day I deepen the breath as often as I can remember to. I have begun to get pretty good at taking brief little breaks to relax and breathe. I use the Flowing Motion whenever I can and try to get in a hundred of them. In the afternoon I take a few moments to use an audio relaxation tape [page 257] to assist in attaining a deep state of relaxation. I have several other practices that I have made up myself. What do you think, doctor," he asked, "am I on the right track?" My response: "Your story is completely inspiring. I am so encouraged when people take action to create their own self-healing program."

Essential Breaths, page 86
Energizing the Organs, page 74

You may want to copy Robert's method for a few days. His routine is an excellent one. You may want to try some of the methods suggested in the next several pages. Or you may simply draw directly from the resources in part 2 to create your own brief and extended practice sessions.

The Momentary Methods

One of the most important aspects of the health enhancement is the ability to remind yourself to activate the healer within frequently throughout the day. Both science and the spiritual traditions confirm the value of being able to return to a state of relaxation often, even in the face of stress. You will discover as you progress in your exploration of personal empowerment and self-healing that the following momentary methods make it possible to reestablish internal peace and self-healing in a very brief period of time.

There is something reassuring about knowing that both the scrutiny of science and the traditions of faith affirm the value of consistently reaching for a state of relaxation.

Use the momentary methods to reclaim your connection with inner strength or intuitive knowing. Two elements can work together through the momentary methods. First, it is useful simply to relax. But it is infinitely more effective when you link relaxation to a second element: having a reason to relax or an attitudinal position that fosters relaxation. Relaxation is enabled when faith and acceptance are present, as discussed in chapter 11.

One of the ancient Qigong methods from China is roughly translated as "Gathering and Cultivating Universal Energies to

Produce a Heavenly Medicine." More literally it translates as "Circulating the Prenatal Universal Elixir in the Energy Channels." The Prenatal Universal is similar to concepts we have explored earlier: "original cause," "the mystery," and "architect of the universe." In this tradition, from ancient Taoism, the practices are based in a "Secret Four-Word Treasure of Success." The four words are *relaxed, tranquil, fearless, carefree.*

The explanation of the "secret" formula for success uses these four words: "Practice the method until the body is relaxed and the mind is tranquil. To attain this state, cultivate the universal wisdom that liberates you to be fearless and carefree." The first two words in the formula, *relaxed* and *tranquil,* suggest the necessary physical state. The second two, *fearless* and *carefree,* suggest the complementary attitudinal and emotional position. Using the "Secret Four-Word Treasure" in every moment and every encounter brings spiritual success, or as Taoism puts it, the practice brings "accumulation of boundless beneficence and virtue." Use the momentary methods to become relaxed, tranquil, fearless, and carefree.

Ten-Second Formulas: Awakening Healing Resources

How long does it take to relax? It seems impossible but the answer is "ten seconds."

First, simply decide to relax. This is a purposeful change of consciousness. Second, take a deep breath. Third, exhale and relax. And that is it. This immediately activates the medicine within you. How could something this simple and this powerful be so easily overlooked? Perhaps it is hard to believe that something so simple could have any value. In addition to shifting your physiology and turning on the healer within, this practice leads to the "accumulation of virtue" according to the ancient source.

You can do this practice frequently throughout the day if you wish. It requires almost no effort whatsoever. Unless you close your eyes during this moment of relaxation, no one will even know that you are doing it. You can even take relaxation breaks in the midst of business meetings or in the company of other people. If you can close your eyes even momentarily, you'll be able to relax even more deeply.

Building on the Ten-Second Formula

As you realize that this moment of relaxation has been beneficial to you, you may decide to extend it. String two or three or
more of these ten-second momentary relaxations together. Five
or six of these ten-second relaxations only take one minute. Try
it. Time yourself.

First, decide to relax. Second, take a deep breath. Give yourself the internal suggestion to relax. Declare internally, "I am
deeply relaxed," or "I am fearless and carefree." Then as you exhale, allow yourself to drift further and further into relaxation. By
the time you reach the end of the exhalation, the whole process
will have taken about ten seconds. Say to yourself, "I promise to
use this wisely." Then return to what you were doing, noticing the
benefits of acting from a position or state of relaxed tranquillity.

You will notice over time that no matter what is happening, remembering to relax will improve your response to the situation.
You may not improve the situation itself by relaxing. But it is guaranteed that you will improve your *reaction* to the situation. Without doing anything you are conserving your energy and protecting
your health just by using this simple momentary self-healing
method. Race-car drivers, basketball players, and even stock mar-
ket analysts will tell you that the "greats" in their field are able to
relax into their work. Eventually, you will become fully aware that
stress and tension never improve anything. The more you practice
this Momentary Method of relaxation, the more deeply you will
understand how tension has been sabotaging you.

An alternative Momentary Method that also takes about ten
seconds starts in exactly the same way. Inhale deeply. When you
begin to exhale, scan your body for areas of tension. Find and release them. You may make a deal with yourself that you will repeat the process (breathing, scanning internally, and releasing
tension) until the whole body feels relaxed.

The first method is simple, the second a little more penetrating in effect. Please feel free to innovate to make this easier for
yourself. If it is more effective for you to use a Sigh of Relief on
the exhalation, then do so. If it is more fun for you or easier to remember to use the ten-second method with the stimulus of some
sort of a reminder, then do that: every hour when the church bell

rings, when the phone rings, at every commercial break during your favorite TV show—your choice.

If you are committed to losing weight, use the Momentary Methods every time you open the cupboard or refrigerator. In stopping smoking or recovering from any negative habit, use the Momentary Methods to remember your goal and reconnect with the wisdom of your choices. If you are in a frustrating or angering situation, use the Momentary Methods to help you communicate honestly.

People often find it useful to associate the Momentary Methods with certain triggers from their work situations. The teachers of young children use recess, lunch, or tense situations to trigger the use of a momentary connection with relaxation and inner wisdom. Nurses frequently use the moment when they are checking blood pressure or pulse or making notes in the patient's chart. Corporate employees use the time between the first and third ring of the phone to take a brief break. Bank tellers use the moment between customers. If you make this simple and fun, the improvement you seek will come easily.

It is impossible to use this simple method too much. If you are seriously ill, using it will help to awaken the healer within you. It will enhance your medical treatment, whether you've chosen conventional medicine, natural medicine, or both. Using the Momentary Methods will enhance drug medicines, herbal medicines, homeopathic medicines, and nutritional supplements. If you are well but want supreme personal vitality, this simple practice will help you to avoid energy drain and increase your base of endurance and resilience.

Ten-Minute Formulas: Feeling Better Fast

You can transform your health future in just a few minutes a day. Draw from all of the self-healing practices to create effective ten-minute sessions. These can be used throughout the day as breaks for those who are working and as recurrent doses of self-healing for those who are not well and are seeking to regain their health.

You are in the best position to devise your own brief sessions because only you are aware of your favorite methods as well as your dislikes and limitations. With the raw material in part 2 you can come up with an almost infinite variety of these brief sessions. The following examples are intended to help you get started and stimulate your creativity. Feel free to innovate. Those who tailor these practices to their own liking are the ones who tend to continue the practice and therefore reach their goal of increased wellness or healing.

Ten-Minute Total-Body Tune-Up

Any or all of these processes may be done lying down, sitting, or standing.

1 Begin by closing your eyes and relaxing. Take five slow, deep, full breaths—exhale audibly, saying, "AHH!" as in a Sigh of Relief.

2 Do the Flowing Motion (page 37) fifteen or twenty times. Adjust the number to fit your situation. Imagine for these few moments that you have nothing to do. Rest in the flow of the motion, imagining that you are a stalk of wheat swaying in a gentle breeze on a beautiful, clear, comfortable summer day.

3 Inhale, interweave the fingers of your right and left hands, raise your arms above your head, palms upward, and reach up toward the ceiling or sky (Reaching Upward, Stretching Outward, page 49). Hold the breath for as long as is comfortable and then exhale slowly through the nose as you bend forward. Honor your comfort zone; do not bend too far. Reach gently down toward the floor, exhaling completely, and wiggle the body gently. Now, slowly return to the upright position in a rolling motion, vertebra by vertebra, and begin again. Repeat three or more times.

4 Vigorously massage both of your ears simultaneously until they feel warm, almost as if they are glowing. This also stimulates reflexes that affect your whole system, particularly the production of beneficial brain chemicals.

5 Allow yourself to relax deeply for a few moments. Initiate a gentle smile by letting the corners of your mouth lift upward ever so slightly. Research has demonstrated that even when you think of smiling, it positively affects your brain chemistry and its connection to the immune system. Notice carefully; you may actually feel this subtle shift occur.

6 Continue with slow, relaxed breaths. Affirm a positive internal message such as "I am grateful for the benefits that I access when

I activate the healer within." Or list a few affirmative thoughts: "Every time I do these practices I help to heal myself (or strengthen my vitality). I purposefully become carefree, knowing that it activates the profound medicine within me. I rest in knowing that these practices initiate automatic physiological processes that have a health-enhancing effect."

7 Acknowledge within that you will sustain the positive effect of this ten-minute session. Reaffirm your willingness to use the Remembering Breath and brief, momentary relaxations frequently throughout the day, especially whenever stress is building.

8 Have a glass of water, juice, or your favorite herbal tea to cleanse and recharge.

Ten-Minute Massage Intensive

1 Vigorously massage your hands and fingers; press and rotate the fingertips. Do your feet and toes too, if time and the situation allow. This stimulates reflexes for all of the organs and glands. Allow your breathing to be full and relaxed (page 61).

2 Vigorously massage both of your ears simultaneously until they feel warm, almost as if they are glowing. This also stimulates reflexes that affect your whole system, particularly the production of beneficial brain chemicals.

3 Massage your left shoulder with your right hand; find the most tense, sore spot and give it a little extra attention (page 69). Simultaneously rotate your head and neck gently. Then massage your right shoulder with your left hand. Next, work on your neck using both hands (page 69). Move your torso around while doing this to get the best effect. Allow your breath to be full but not urgent.

4 Do some massage of the abdomen and colon, combined with abdominal breathing. On the exhalation, as the abdomen contracts inward, press in with extended fingers held close together. Apply a penetrating, mildly rotary motion. Bend forward. Seek areas that seem tense or knotted and knead them gently (page 72).

5 Place the palm of one hand on or near the part of your body that is the most uncomfortable or the least able to do its job. Place the palm of your other hand over your second most painful or deficient part. Now, move about, stretch, or wiggle around

gently (page 80). The most important healing resource is within you. You are working this resource into areas where it has been unable to penetrate, just as you use penetrating oil to loosen a rusty bolt or screw. Imagine or feel, if you can, heat and healing energy passing from your hands into your body. Allow the breath to be full and relaxed. Add Sighs of Relief to enhance the effect.

6 Place your hands in your lap or allow them to dangle at your sides if you are standing. Notice the sensations within. This is your internal medicine working. Remember, it is a subtle sensation, and even if you do not feel it, the effect is still present.

7 Have a glass of water, some fruit, or vegetable juice or your favorite herbal tea to cleanse and recharge your system.

Ten-Minute Movement Series

String the following movements together in a series where you flow from one movement to the next. This is exactly the idea in the Chinese practice called Taiji (Tai Chi). Instead of 108 movements as in Taiji, this series is much briefer, and you can change it around as much as you want. There is no particular way to make the transition to the next movement; use your imagination.

1 Carefully initiate the Preliminary Posture (page 35). Just rest in this position for a few moments. Allow yourself to slow down, turn your attention inward, and agree to keep your mind clear of lists, concerns, and details.

2 Begin the Flowing Motion (page 37). Do ten to twenty repetitions. Feel yourself flowing into a deep state of relaxation.

3 Without stopping, shift to the Right and Left Bending of the Spine (page 40). Choose an appropriate number of repetitions; deeply relax. If it is comfortable, bring the arm on the side that is stretching up over the head.

4 Gently transition to the Front and Back Bending of the Spine (page 44). Remember to add the contraction of the perineum muscles deep in the pelvis, as well as contract the toes, eyes, and face and press the fists together in front. Then completely relax as you bend in the opposite direction and look upward between the hands. Do an appropriate number of repetitions. Then transition gently to the next movement.

5 Interlace the fingers and commence several repetitions of Reaching Upward, Stretching Outward (page 49). Lift up onto your toes if you can do so comfortably. Continue to relax.

6 Do the Spontaneous Movement method (page 51) for a few moments, and then add Connecting the Spots massage (page 80). Remember that placing the hands in this way mobilizes energy that may be blocked and helps to release tension or pain.

7 Conclude in the Preliminary Posture with a few deep breaths. In China a typical ending for a practice session includes relaxing in this posture with the hands one on top of the other on or just below the navel. This area is called the Tan Tien, which roughly means the place where the inner medicine accumulates. Literally it means "heavenly elixir field."

The ten-second and ten-minute formulas are like the trim on the house of health that you are building. You will begin to realize that there are places here and there in your day when you can add them in. They modify and enhance the power of your self-healing program. Notice that the ten-second methods can fit in almost anywhere. As you realize the power of the ten-minute formulas, you will be inspired to place them carefully in your life as well.

Nurse Jan's Story

Jan is an incredible nurse. Just ask anybody who has experienced her expertise. She has worked in the innovative, multidisciplinary pain management program and the birthing center at one of Santa Barbara's hospitals. Or you could ask the hundreds of people she has served through the parish nursing program or through her years as a massage therapist and Yoga instructor. Jan believes that the greatest source of healing is "God and a good laugh." She feels that the most important health care consists of the self-healing practices. She is particularly skilled at modifying and adapting the practices for herself and others in order to keep the process interesting and fun. Here is her story:

I have a tremendous respect for medicine. It pulled me through a difficult string of accidents. I was always super-healthy. Then I had a car accident where I was thrown out of the car at sixty miles an hour and then hit by a truck. At first there was no alternative to the medical treatment, which patched me up and probably saved my life. Then, during an emergency delivery at the birth center I had a second strain to my back, which complicated my case. There was a point in my treatment where it was obvious that medicine had reached its limit.

I could have been paralyzed. I guess I'm a little like a stuntwoman. Massage and chiropractic have been helpful, but you can't have treatment every day and that's what I needed. I am averse to using pain medication after having so many experiences with people in the pain center who not only had the torment of the pain itself but also dependence on pain medication. So I had to figure out how to treat myself. I've tried thousands of techniques.

I have symptoms, particularly pain and discomfort, but they don't undermine my joy. I am not interested in being disabled. I am constantly participating and enjoying. I do lots of walking. Variety is my key. Variety in work, variety in play, and variety in my self-healing practice. After years of doing and teaching Yoga I had to modify it because of my condition. Special breathing exercises are my first line of defense because I can do them anywhere.

Because of my nature, I have to adapt my personal practice so that it fits into my life and has lots of variety. I don't set aside a single chunk of time to practice. I prefer to incorporate self-healing throughout the day. With walks, the deep breathing, numerous brief stops for some gentle movements or the Gathering Breath, occasional momentary check-ins, lots of self-massage (I move around on a carpeted area and position tennis balls to apply pressure), and some deep relaxation to music I probably end up doing nearly an hour of practice integrated throughout my day.

Remembering Breath (page 89)
Flowing Motion (page 37)
Gathering Breath (page 96)
Momentary Method (page 122)

Self-Applied Massage (page 55)
Deep Relaxation (page 99)

Jan goes on: "Two major themes in my self-healing are faith and humor. Since I was a child I have had a very personal relationship with God, nature, and the universe. Along with my health enhancement practices I am prayerful and grateful. Plus, laughter always reduces my discomfort. I understand through the medical literature that laughing triggers the production of pain-reducing brain chemicals. I may actually be experiencing symptoms, but it's almost like I have a protective shield of faith and laughter."

Jan has led our Wednesday Self-Healing Practice Session many times. Participants are pleased with her focus on humor, spirit, variety, and self-acceptance. She tells them, "Don't ever compare yourself with anyone; it can only lead to useless pride or painful shame. Don't compare your health enhancement program to anyone else's; it is a good sign that yours is different, since everyone has different needs. Don't even compare yourself to yourself. Every day you are different; allow for that, celebrate that."

Jan's set of practices for the Wednesday sessions is similar to her usual routine. However, she is always changing it, adding music and stimulating laughter. She has found that the same practices have been useful in her work with the church parishes as well. Here's how she describes these sessions:

First, we do a momentary, full-body check-in. I call it a freeze-frame. It takes just a moment. We begin with a deep, slow breath. On the exhalation we scan the whole body for tension. The goal is to learn how to notice now and then, using the freeze-frame, where we accumulate tension. Is your stress location always the same, or is it different? You can learn from this.

Then we do several gentle body practices. I particularly like the Flowing Motion because you can do it anywhere. You can do it sitting, or you can modify it so you can do it in public. Shrink it, so you raise up just a little on your toes and just barely move your hands and then just slightly lift your toes. It's fun to do, it's like your little secret, and you can visualize that you are doing big extravagant movements even though you are hardly moving at all. Watch how turning your attention to this practice changes your posture and your breathing—it's great.

I also like the Gathering Breath because it combines the breathing and movement. It is like gathering in light or heavenly essence; it has a spiritual feel to me. Then we do self-massage and I always demonstrate using tennis balls. You just lie down, usually on a carpeted area. Using a tennis ball you can work on spots in the back or hips that otherwise you would have to pay fifty or seventy-five dollars to have a massage practitioner work on for you. We usually do hand and ear and shoulder self-massage as well.

We end with relaxation to soothing music and guided imagery. The music helps the mind to move out of the thought realm. We visualize that our legs are like straws dipped into earth, the top of our heads are like a radio-wave antenna. On the inhalations we pull in healing resources, and on the exhalations we circulate those resources to the organs. Before we end, we send energy to others. It's kind of like praying but also like sending love or gratitude.

The design of the practice always changes because I like variety. If it varies, then it's fun for me, and if it's fun for me, then I'm humorous and enthusiastic. Laughter and enthusiasm are contagious; they cause people to want to continue the practices.

Momentary Method (page 122)
Flowing Motion (page 37)
Gathering Breath (page 96)
Massage with tennis balls
Massaging the Hands (page 61)
Massaging the Ears (page 65)
Massaging the Shoulders (page 68)
One of the relaxation and meditation methods (page 99)

"I love the work of teaching and empowering people," Jan concludes, "especially the elders and those who are unwell. There is so much wisdom in our elders; it's sorrowful that we don't honor and respect the elders now like we did in ancient cultures. I am delighted to participate in motivating and empowering people. Because of my own pain I am very suited to teach people with pain and disease. When I tell my story, they wonder how I am even alive. The fact that I am active and laughing allows them to believe that they can be too.

"Funny thing, it has become obvious to me that my medical degree and training give me license to do this work. But it is my personal history and my personal self-healing practice that are the real credentials that help people to heal."

CHAPTER 9

Deepening Your Practice

Nothing is more encouraging than the unquestionable human capacity to consciously refine and elevate life.

Henry David Thoreau,
transcendental philosopher
and citizen activist

BECAUSE YOU ARE IN A PROCESS OF IMPROVEMENT THAT could serve you for the rest of your life, it is not actually important whether your daily practice is fully perfected now. Feel free to start anywhere, with the idea that you will be continuously improving, exploring, and correcting your course in both the near and far future. In my own personal practice of these methods I have been through hundreds of stages. During certain periods I have changed and learned new methods every few days. At other times I have continued with a similar set of practices for several months and even years at a stretch. Almost every day I still practice a form of Taiji (Tai Chi) that I first learned more than twenty years ago.

Most people love variation. For many years as a part of the Health Action Clinic program we have held a one-hour practice session every Wednesday at 11 A.M. Generally, the weekly routine followed the same order as the practices in part 2: movement, self-massage, breathing practices, and deep relaxation. Frequently, I would be called out of town to lecture or do some consulting at hospitals around the country. In order to be consistent we had a number of substitute instructors who would bring their own personal approach to self-healing to the one-hour session.

Human nature is so diverse and fascinating. When a different routine was introduced by these guest facilitators, there were always a handful of the regular practitioners who were excited and pleased with the change. Typically, another handful would complain that they didn't like the change. What's more, over time it was not the same people who did or didn't like the change.

Everyone is different. Our likes, dislikes, limitations, and even our moods are always changing. In life it is best to be willing to enjoy change by being flexible while gently sustaining some of our preferences. In the learning and practicing of self-healing, the same is true. Certainly, you'll want to clarify and pursue your preferences, but also foster your willingness to embrace variety. Try lots of different approaches, time frames, and methods in your quest to refine and elevate life.

Extended Formulas: Medicine for the Sick, Insurance for the Well

The firm foundation of your vitality and of your personal health improvement program is the extended practice session that you will eventually want to place carefully in your day. The Momentary and Ten-Minute Methods are the trim on your house of health, longevity, and empowerment. The extended practice that we are about to explore is the house itself. Extended practice is your guarantee of enduring health for your body, which is the temple of your self, your mind and spirit.

Athletes and health enthusiasts frequently spend several hours a day seeking fitness. Their house of health is generally quite strong. Health trainers, Yoga teachers, aerobics instructors, and other professionals in the wellness field suggest that fitness practice should last from forty to sixty minutes at least every other day. My own experiences and those of the many people with whom I have worked have demonstrated that it is actually easier to do the practices every day.

To designate and then open up the time for your practice will require some prioritizing. It's actually pretty easy if you just ask the question, "What do I want?" If you are sick and the answer is "I want to be well," then you have just prioritized taking action to implement an extended self-healing session on a regular basis. If you are well and the answer is "I want more energy, clarity, and productivity," then you have just prioritized an extended session of energy-enhancing practice on a regular basis.

Most people think immediately, "I can't spare that time." But "I want to be well" and "I can't spare that time" are two very different priority statements. It may take a while to find your true priorities, so be kind to yourself. Beware, however: more than just a few of the patients I have seen for acupuncture and herbal medicine have noted with hindsight, "I wish I had taken better care before my health got so out of hand." Once you have lost your health, you are guaranteed to have to put forth additional effort to regain it.

You may want to start with a practice session every other day. Or you may want to work with just twenty minutes every day for a while. Most people, however, find that at twenty minutes they are really just getting started. When you use your personal experience as your guide, you will get direct feedback from internal wisdom and intuition that will direct your practice. Everybody is different, so you will have to pay attention. Follow the guidelines from page 26. Don't do too much, and don't leave your comfort zone. Have fun, go slow, experiment and innovate, turn your attention inward for feedback. You will literally feel the healing resources circulating and interacting within. You will learn how to add here and there and when to take a break or cut back.

In the parks in China, the average practice session is sixty minutes. Many people do special practices that last over an hour. And many do abbreviated sessions for personal reasons. Once I followed a man for a while who was in his hospital pajamas; the hospital was right by the park. He was doing the cancer recovery walking method, with the *xi, xi, hu* breathing (page 93). He walked slowly in the stylized, self-healing way to a small lake. He did a brief set of self-healing practices by the lake and then did the walking method back to the hospital. It was obvious that he was not well. His practice lasted twenty-five to thirty minutes.

In the Purple Bamboo Park in Beijing there is a group that practices for three hours each day. Master Shi, the teacher, is famous for his skill. He declares, "Practice is necessary to achieve harmony, which is the balance of heaven's energy and earth's energy. This leads to health and vitality. This heals disease and resolves conflict." During the three-hour practice session, Master Shi's students practice meditation and Taiji.

Everyone will eventually learn how to design his or her own most effective practice. It is not hard. It just requires your willingness to pay attention. These methods can also be mixed with any other fitness program, including walking, swimming, dancing, and even aerobics or weight training. As I've said, the Chinese believe that mild activity done in a state of deep relaxation has a greater beneficial effect than more vigorous exercises, and they apply this belief to their self-healing practices. But if you bring the intention to relax to your practice of walking, swimming, or low-impact aerobics, these activities too can become a kind of Qigong (Chi Kung) practice.

Outside of Asia it is typically believed, unfortunately, that fitness practice is impossible or impractical for people who are severely ill, particularly if they are restricted to a bed or chair. Actually, this is not true. There are no barriers to the use of these self-healing practices. In cases where the illness is quite severe, the practices can be modified. For example, patients (students) who are paralyzed or incapacitated can imagine they are doing the practices. Research has shown that the brain cannot tell the difference between imagined activity and actual activity. When you dream of running to catch a bus, many of the biological characteristics of physical exertion are triggered in the body even though you are actually asleep.

Even when one is not severely ill, it is still better to limit strenuous exercise and use just the self-healing practices until a foundation of vitality is secure. According to both the Chinese Qigong experts and the Indian Yoga experts, it is best to build more vigorous exercise into the fitness routine only after health has been recovered. In those who are well, however, mixing conventional fitness exercises with self-healing methods is quite reasonable.

The Wednesday SAHEM Practice Session

One variation of a one-hour set of daily practices evolved over time at our Wednesday practice session. We conducted this session weekly for three years at the Health Action Clinic and for another three years at one of the Santa Barbara Parks and Recreation facilities. People would come a little early or would linger afterward if they liked to mix socially. You might want to try this practice set yourself a few times as a starting place for your own extended personal practice.

Start with a few repetitions of the gentle movement methods. Begin immediately to try to recognize when you have done enough and transition to the next part of the practice. This requires being attentive. It is easy for the mind to wander off into all sorts of busyness. An important aspect of these practices is to calm and direct the mind. Noticing what is happening within is a useful assignment for the mind during your practice time. The Chinese suggest seeking a "mental neutral" state—or even the state of "cheerful indifference." The latter is the marvelous ability to be happy and unconcerned at the same time, kind of like being happy about nothing.

First do the Flowing Motion, followed by the Right and Left Bending of the Spine and the Front and Back Bending of the Spine. Next do Tracing the Acupuncture Energy Channels, which transitions into Energizing the Organs and then to Massaging the Abdomen. All of these can be done standing. If you or the person you are teaching is limited to a wheelchair or bed, you can adapt these movements accordingly.

The breath is always full and relaxed. Direct the mind to something simple. Notice what you are experiencing internally. Try to sense the activity of the biological processes within you. Monitor carefully for signs that you may be doing too much, particularly if you are dealing with a difficult disease challenge. Resist making lists, worrying, or thinking about things that you should have done or that you wish you had not done. Research shows that a calm mind triggers the best of the medicine within.

Then sit in a chair. A dining table chair, desk chair, folding chair, or stool is best. Comfy chairs, chairs that you sink into, and armchairs will restrict your ability to do the practices efficiently. Continue now with your practice by massaging each of the hands in turn. Feel for the sore points and give them extra attention. Then massage both ears simultaneously until they are glowing and warm. Now, massage the left shoulder with the right hand and then the right shoulder with the left hand. Next, work on both sides of the neck with your fingertips extended and held together. As always the breath is full and relaxed.

Continue with five to seven repetitions of the Gathering Breath (page 96). Finally, select one of the relaxation practices from chapter 7.

Flowing Motion (page 37)
Right and Left Bending of the Spine (page 40)
Front and Back Bending of the Spine (page 44)
Tracing the Acupuncture Energy Channels (page 70)
Energizing the Organs (page 74)
Massaging the Abdomen (page 72)
Massaging the Hands (page 61)
Massaging the Ears (page 65)
Massaging the left shoulder with the right hand and then the
     right shoulder with the left hand (page 69)
Massaging both sides of the neck with extended fingertips
     (page 69)
Five to seven repetitions of the Gathering Breath (page 96)
One of the relaxation practices from chapter 7 (pages 99 to 110)

We have used this set of practices, with minor changes, for over six years. If you want to use a formula that is "tried and true," then be assured that this set of practices has been used by thousands of the people with whom we have worked. However, following a particular formula for your practice does not guarantee the greatest benefit. The greatest benefit will be gained by finding the unique set of practices that fit together for you and create a sense of well-being. Using your chosen practices vigilantly over time will heal and empower you.

Daily Program

Most of the people who have integrated self-healing into their lives will tell you that sooner or later they realized that they needed to make a special place in their lives every day for the practice of health enhancement methods. Life is complex and demanding, and our relationship with time is mysterious. You already know that it is challenging to find time. You also know that if you wait until you get some time, it will never happen. It is impossible, really, either to "find time" or "get time." Oddly enough, however, it is possible to *allow* time. Or you can *take* time. You can even, through a kind of magic, *make* time. The magic comes through honestly prioritizing and then telling the truth to the people in your life about your priorities. Philosophers will tell you that you can alter time with your attitudes. "Time flies when we are having fun," as the old saying goes.

Many of the people who have learned and practiced the self-healing methods feel that their practice time becomes special personal time, even sacred time. Busy people typically report that the practices give them a period of quiet in which to unwind, rest, and recharge their weary bodies and minds. They find that the practices enhance their intuition, their adaptability to stress, and their creativity. I have worked with several hospital administrators who have said, "How can I expect to improve the health care system if I haven't yet understood how to improve my own health?" The human resources director of one of the major aircraft manufacturing companies said recently, "We are realizing that it is impossible to improve our productivity further without giving our employees permission to improve themselves."

People who are very sick automatically have time; they are not at work or at school. And because the self-healing methods can be altered to fit each case, a very sick person can do a mild form of self-healing practice almost constantly throughout the day. The Remembering Breath, the In, In, Out breath *(xi, xi, hu)*, and the Momentary Methods are ways to do the practices anywhere—at work, at play, at school, even in bed.

Once a Day

For most of the people who have been doing these practices seriously to regain health or to sustain health and increase vitality, a daily session has become typical. Those who are deriving maximum benefit have generally progressed to forty to sixty minutes of practice per day. For many who are just getting started, the period of time may be shorter and less frequent. Either way is perfect. The primary issue is to have the process be appropriate, beneficial, and fun. You can change it anytime. In fact, you will definitely change it as you progress, learn, and evolve.

I like to use these practices at the beginning of the day. Usually, I practice for about one hour. I am very fortunate to live within walking distance of exquisite natural settings, so I practice outside almost always. The color of the dawn, the sound of waves against the shore, the changing seasons are all part of the healing for me. On rainy days or when I lecture away from home, I do the practices indoors. In China and in major cities around the United States, I use the public parks.

In China, several million people do these practices every day. Usually people's practice lasts about an hour. The Chinese suggest that these practices be done in the early morning when night is transitioning to day and the dew is still on the grass. The shift from night to day is considered a special time as light replaces darkness and the effect of rest is fresh.

On a recent trip to China's Huang Mountains, I decided to find a special spot where I could watch the sun rise and practice some Qigong. When I got to the place I was amazed to find over a thousand people there ahead of me. When the sun peaked over the horizon, everyone sighed or cheered, enthusiastically greeting the light of a new day.

Twice or More a Day

When it is possible or necessary, two practice sessions can be better than one. For the individual who is unwell and interested in accelerating healing, two practice sessions are useful. If the individual is weak or fatigues easily, two short sessions are better than one long session. For people who are busy, it may be necessary to practice in two shorter sessions—one in the morning to get things going and one in the evening to slow things down.

For those who are particularly challenged by some health problem, it may be better to do numerous short sessions throughout the day. Recall that Jan, the registered nurse whom we met earlier, uses breath practice along with stretching and self-massage throughout the day to relieve pain. Bob, the physicist from Virginia, uses his list of 107 activities to trigger his use of the Remembering Breath nearly a hundred times a day. At numerous hospitals throughout China where people with incurable diseases go to recover their health, the practice of Qigong is frequently spread throughout the whole day.

When and How More Is Better, When and How More Is Worse

Generally, with these very gentle self-healing practices the more you can practice the better. The naturally occurring self-healing mechanisms are always operating within the human system. The blood circulates, oxygen and nutritional elements migrate to the cells, the lymph facilitates the elimination of waste products, the chemistry of the brain and neurological systems coordinate millions of functions and interactions among the body's seventy-five trillion cells.

When disease or pain appears, it is a sign that the system has become deficient, dysfunctional, or out of harmony. Function that is usually ample and organized has become deficient and disorganized. If one is alert to and aware of dysfunction early in the process, a small amount of health enhancement activity can set the system right; this is that "ounce of prevention." If one is less alert and less aware of the dysfunction until it has become severe, then a larger amount of health enhancement activity—a "pound of cure"—will be required.

In either case, self-healing methods can help to rehabilitate the function of the system. By increasing the intention to improve health and then using self-applied health enhancement methods, the natural activity of the blood, lymph, brain chemistry, and all the natural healing systems within the body are increased. Whether these self-healing methods are used with or without medical intervention, they will increase the natural activities within that can improve your health.

In certain severe cases, however, self-healing methods can tax the system. In severe cases of cancer, multiple sclerosis, and chronic fatigue syndrome, the practice of very gentle health-enhancing methods can definitely help to restore health. However, they must be implemented carefully. Up to a certain threshold the practices are restorative; this is what we have been calling the comfort zone. Past this point continued practice can be detrimental. This is frequently called "too much of a good thing."

Research has shown that when an individual crosses the anaerobic threshold, there is a dramatic disabling of the immune system, which then requires an extended period of time to recover (a more detailed account of the anaerobic threshold may be found in the phsysiology section of the appendix). In serious disease there may be a limit as to how much exercise a person can do before crossing this threshold. Dozens of people—particularly those with chronic fatigue, HIV, and myofascitis—whom I have seen clinically, who thought that vigorous exercise should help them to heal, have been surprised to find themselves incapacitated after small amounts of brisk activity.

The threshold of the comfort zone, if carefully honored, will expand. A great example of this happened with a patient who had scleroderma. She became overly enthusiastic in her early use of the health enhancement practices and caused several brief setbacks. When she learned to pay careful attention to her limits, however, her endurance and vitality improved, and she was able to achieve a complete remission from the disease. Those who modify their practice to honor the comfort zone can create miracles. The key is to pay very close attention during the practice as well as afterward.

One of the people from the Cancer Recovery Society whom I met in China made this point while the group was having tea after their practice session. She reported that when she was originally visited by one of the members of the Cancer Recovery Society, she was unable to get out of the hospital bed. She became so enthusiastic after hearing several of the testimonials of recovering cancer patients (students) that she attempted to do the *xi, xi, hu* (In, In, Out breath, page 93) all day long. She found that when she did it too much she became fatigued. Eventually, with careful modification, she found the proper amount of practice. It is her theory that when she found the right timing and amount for the practice, that every ensuing practice session contributed to her recovery. On the day that she told this story she was celebrating the seventh-year anniversary of her recovery process since the diagnosis of stomach cancer.

Because the practices are gentle, the worst that will occur if you overdo will be a need for extra rest. Rest is one of our most powerful self-healing tools. When the body asks for rest—when we feel tired, fatigued, or exhausted—we need to give it rest. Rest is a potent medicine. Coffee and soda are not medicine. The goal in severe disease is to find the right amount of practice so that you get the acceleration of natural self-healing activities without doing too much and canceling the benefit. Finding the stop sign at the edge of the comfort zone is the key. You can do this by establishing a new habit of paying attention to subtle signs and signals from the healer within.

Do what seems to be less than enough of the practices on a frequent basis throughout the day. Then expand on this amount slowly. Using this process, most people discover where the threshold of overexertion is without ever leaving the comfort zone. Don't compare yourself to others; don't even compare yourself to yourself. Notice that the threshold changes every day. Notice that nourishing the habit of being attentive within and deepening your awareness bring improvement surely and slowly.

Continuous Practice

If the most profound medicine is produced within us and if it is easy to activate it, then why wouldn't we stay connected to the process of producing this marvelous resource continuously? In actuality, you are continuously producing natural healing resources within you. After all, how did you sustain your vitality throughout your life? We rarely ask, "What causes and sustains our life and our health?" This miracle, the "original cause" of life and health, the healer within, has been serving you spontaneously for decades.

However, as we have discussed, the natural self-healing capacity can become deficient, or blocked, or imbalanced through injury, unhealthy circumstances, or disease. The health enhancement and self-healing methods are powerful tools that can be used to reestablish strength, flow, and harmony in our internal mechanisms of self-healing. It may not be possible to do body movement, self-massage, or deep meditation continuously. However, you can sprinkle them throughout your day. And it is possible to take deep breaths on a regular basis, as described in the Remembering Breath (page 89). It is also possible to engage in the Momentary Methods (page 122) throughout the day.

Plus, there is another, deeper level of practice that you may want to explore. At this level the focus is to sustain a continuous connection with the source or force that is the "original cause" of the spontaneous activity of the healer within. "Original cause" is a way of describing the origins from which the architect of the universe created the human experience. In the Western world we usually use the word *God*. The ancients in every culture have such a word. In India it is Atma. In China it is called Mystery or the Prenatal Origin. Continuous self-healing practice can be accomplished by sustaining direct awareness of the source of all the gifts, blessings, and promises of the spiritual traditions—the original cause.

Recall the "Secret Four-Word Formula for Success" (page 123) from the ancient Chinese Taoist tradition—relaxed, tranquil, fearless, carefree? Unceasing awareness of this formula, sustained throughout the day, is a potent method for continuous practice. Some traditions repeat the "names of God" as continuous practice. In the Christian tradition a formula for continuous practice was given: "pray unceasingly." Reaching for continuous practice is a doorway leading from self-healing to spiritual practice.

Modifications for Hospital Bed or Wheelchair

The most significant modifications of the self-healing methods are necessary when the individual using them is incapacitated. In cases where individuals are extremely ill, incapacitated by paralysis or injury, or near death, or they have recently experienced surgery, the self-healing methods will need to be changed significantly.

The Hospital Bed

When you are limited to bed yourself or are working with someone who is, the self-healing methods can be easily adapted. Carla from Virginia reported recently that she used the self-healing methods from my video *Awakening and Mastering the Medicine Within* (page 257) before and after serious colon surgery. Before the operation she used the practices to prepare herself, to reduce the trauma of the procedure, and to speed up and improve the postoperative period.

Following the surgery she used the practices to accelerate healing and recovery. When she could not move from her bed, she continued to practice. "When I couldn't move I just visualized doing the practices. I also simply watched the video. I was amazed. Both imagining doing the practices and viewing the video gave me a definite sense of well-being, as if I had actually done them. In addition, I was able to begin using the breathing methods almost immediately after the surgery."

When it is impossible to move, start with the breathing. The Essential Breath becomes the Remembering Breath when it is used consciously over time. The In, In, Out breath *(xi, xi hu)* is often used in China by recovering cancer patients who are students of self-healing. The breathing pumps the lymph, which activates the elimination of waste products from the system. This is a critical aspect of the healer within.

When it is impossible to move, use the deep relaxation methods and imagine doing the body movements. Relaxation causes the internal chemistry to shift into self-healing activity. In a deep state of relaxation, the immune system is at its most active. Fear, worry, and anxiety tend to interrupt the natural healing within. Visualizing doing the gentle body movements triggers many of the same internal mechanisms that the movements themselves activate.

An individual who cannot move can actually do quite a bit of self-healing practice. A family member or nurse can do some of the massage methods, particularly the massaging of the feet, which is a very effective healing practice. In the 1960s and 1970s when I had my first experiences working in hospitals I worked the night shift. I gained some notoriety among the nurses for helping to decrease the patients' need for sleep and pain medicines. When my duties as a patient attendant were complete, I would get requests from the head nurse to visit the patients who were in pain or struggling with insomnia. I simply used the foot rubbing method described in chapter 5 and a modification of the hand motions from the Gathering Breath from chapter 6. This second method, which is very common in China, is called energy healing (Qigong healing). It has recently become popular with the nursing community and is called Therapeutic Touch.

As in the Gathering Breath, the hands do not actually touch the body. After massaging the feet I would pass my hands near the patient's body at a distance of about three inches and "unruffle" areas where I felt heat, cold, or a kind of energy tangle. I was amazed at how effective this method was; frequently the patient would fall asleep with no medication. Nurses at hospitals in Ohio, California, and Hawaii called it hocus-pocus, but they all requested that I continue. This was one of the experiences that inspired me to study Chinese medicine.

Once you or the person you are working with has become able to move the fingers or toes, then focus on movements with the breathing. When it is possible to do larger movements, then begin to adapt the Flowing Motion, the arm movements from the Front and Back Bending of the Spine, and the arm movements from Reaching Upward, Stretching Outward. When the practice calls for lifting the weight of the body up onto the toes, just stretch the toes away from the body. When the practice calls for lifting the toes, then flex the toes toward the head.

As soon as it is possible, move the practice into a chair.

The Chair or Wheelchair

Many of the people who have benefited the most from the self-healing methods have started the practice sitting for numerous reasons. Some use the chair practices because they want to practice while at their desk at work, or watching TV, or listening to the radio. Others have had to do the practices sitting because of illness, pain, injury, or weakness. Some were elders who had become so fearful of falling that they had become very sedentary.

One multiple sclerosis patient began her practices in her wheelchair. Soon she felt confident enough to do the practices standing while holding onto the chair when necessary. Another, who had polio as a child, would start the practices standing and then sit when she became fatigued. In several of the corporations that have provided training in the methods, we have taught people to practice sitting. This helps relieve stress and increase productivity for people whose work occurs at desks.

At the Wednesday Self-Healing Practice Session numerous participants, especially those with severe fatigue, have done the whole session sitting in order to conserve energy. When we did a special eight-week series in the self-healing practices that was linked to the senior lunch program sponsored by the Area Agencies on Aging in southern California, a number of the participants started out sitting but gained enough strength over eight weeks to end the program doing the gentle body movements standing.

Except for the gentle movement practices, most of the methods—self-massage, breath practice, and deep relaxation—can be done without modification in a sitting position. To begin to build vitality, endurance, and balance, start by doing the movement practices sitting if you wish. Later graduate to standing practice. The most important rule for those who are older or who are unwell is to go slowly and resist doing too much. Those who feel they may fall should build up their strength before doing the standing methods. One excellent study of Taiji demonstrated that it improves balance and reduces falls. The practices will eventually give you back your balance. Don't rush to get there too soon; instead, relax to get there well. That is what "slow but sure" is all about.

When sitting to do the movements, you will find it easier (although not absolutely necessary) to use a stool or a chair without arms. When in a wheelchair, adapt the movements to avoid the arms of the chair, unless they can be removed temporarily. When the description of the movement asks you to lift the weight of the body on the toes, lift your heels as high as you can. When the description asks for you to rest on your heels, raise your toes as high as you can. Again, remember that building up slowly to expand your comfort zone is better than racing to break through and then feeling like you have overdone it.

Working with Your Doctor

Health care used to be based on treating people after they had lost their health. True health care is based on keeping people well. Formerly the doctor held the key. Now you hold the key. Your ability to operate within the three areas of choice we have discussed—attitudes, lifestyle, and self-care—determine whether your personal health care system is a success or a failure.

With the self-applied health enhancement methods as your tools, your self-care capability is advanced. With a moderate daily practice of health enhancement and self-healing methods you are likely to maintain a high level of health and vitality. Mild health challenges will be easily handled through your self-healing practice. However, it is unlikely that we will magically shift to a perfect new health care system overnight. So there are a number of important questions to answer regarding self-healing, medical treatment, and interaction with the physician community.

When a wellness-based health care system is working well, when is a doctor or medical treatment needed? Accidents, injuries, and medical problems are not likely to disappear in the near future. While it is true that over 70 percent of disease is preventable, we have a lot of improving to do before we reach that point. Until that day, the health enhancement methods will be a powerful complement to medical treatment when it is necessary. And even when that day comes, the remaining 30 percent of today's diseases may still be a problem, so an interaction between medical treatment and self-care will always be prevalent.

Should one wait to be told by a doctor to practice self-healing and health enhancement? No. In fact, it is best to learn to practice these methods as a child. They will become a practical part of one's daily life if learned from a friend, a parent, a grandparent, or a teacher. Experts in child development feel that the formative period for life habits is in the first seven years of a child's life. When children learn the self-healing methods in their early years, their approach to doctors, hospitals, and medical treatment as adults will be completely different from the old twentieth-century system of disease care.

Is it important to have a specific disease or diagnosis before beginning to use the methods? As we have discussed, it is best to learn these practices while one is well in order to avoid disease. Begin your practice now. When ill health occurs, which will be less likely because of your practice, then accelerate your use of the methods. In a disease-based system it is necessary to work with a clearly defined disorder; treatment, then, must be consistent with the diagnosis. However, the self-healing methods are the same for all diseases and all diagnoses.

Do the self-healing and health enhancement methods eliminate one's need for a physician? The ideal answer is yes. However, in many cases a complementary relationship will exist between medical intervention and self-healing. The perfect health care system is a holistic interaction between wellness (health maintenance and promotion), natural medicine, and conventional medicine. This means that in an ideal system, you may interact with a health promotion counselor or wellness educator along with one or several doctors of conventional medicine and natural healing. Or you might interact with a doctor of conventional medicine along with a massage practitioner or a teacher of Yoga or Qigong. In different communities the makeup of multidisciplinary health improvement teams is diverse in order to meet various situations most effectively. Some people will spontaneously attain supreme wellness with little or no medical support. Others will improve health or manage disease with assistance from health facilitators, teachers, and physicians.

How does one know when to seek a doctor? In certain health care plans, each person has a primary care doctor who keeps track of his or her basic health level. In these cases either a doctor or a primary care clinical associate (nurse practitioner or physician assistant) provides annual or occasional health checkups. In other cases, people choose to be more on their own through self-care. In either situation, it is always appropriate to increase the level of self-care activity when health problems arise. Check any rapid-onset health problem with a conventional or holistic physician immediately. If increasing your self-healing activities does not seem to resolve the health challenge or increase your well-being, you have, in a sense, made a general self-diagnosis of a problem or physical imbalance that would benefit from a doctor's assistance. See your physician soon, and review your lifestyle for ways to improve your self-healing plan.

What kind of doctor should one seek? Because there is a natural healer within us that produces a powerful natural medicine, it is only logical to seek a doctor who deals with methods that accelerate these natural healing energies. In most cases some variety of massage or body therapy along with gentle herbal formulas will stimulate a natural healing response and reestablish internal harmony. The next level of attention would be with either a conventional primary care physician or with an acupuncturist, osteopath, chiropractor, naturopath, or homeopath. In many cases it is best to see one of these natural healing doctors in conjunction with the services of your primary care physician. In a comprehensive and integrated medical system, the primary care and natural healing practitioners cooperate to help you understand when and if surgery or drug therapy is a reasonable alternative.

Is there any situation where self-healing should be replaced by medical treatment only? No. Even in accidents, injuries, surgical cases, and severe diseases the use of the self-healing methods will complement the medical treatment and speed recovery. While you are in the ambulance, preparing for a surgery, having a broken bone set, or undergoing surgery or chemotherapy—practice the self-healing methods. After the broken bone is set, after the surgery, after the chemotherapy, between physician visits, between doses of medication, between acupuncture treatments, massages, or osteopathic manipulation—practice the methods. Along with herbs, vitamins, special diets, homeopathic remedies—practice self-healing.

Margaret's Story

Margaret was diagnosed with chronic lymphocytic leukemia (CLL) in 1987. This disease consists of an abnormal increase in white blood cells that is considered to be a kind of cancer, as it is characterized by uncontrolled and unnatural cell growth. Her doctor informed her that CLL generally worsens slowly and that there was no medical treatment that would retard the progression of the disorder. However, he stated, medical treatment including both chemotherapy and radiation would be available when complications such as swollen lymph nodes, an enlarged spleen, or restricted breathing became a problem.

Relieved to know that the progress of the disease would be slow and alarmed that there was no medical solution, Margaret began to explore alternative strategies for health enhancement. She looked into nutritional and herbal support, and she began to practice some self-healing methods. Here is Margaret's story.

I began to refine my diet, use vitamin and herbal supplements, and become more focused with my exercise and self-care practices. An inner, almost spiritual kind of intuition directed me. I felt that anything I would do to increase my health generally would slow the progress of the disease. My physician did not confirm this idea, but it felt right to me. I had gained tremendous support from prayer and the study material from my church over the years, so I deepened my spiritual practice as well.

I was always a healthy person overall so I didn't really expect to feel much different. I did have a sense of well-being, particularly when I did my self-healing practices. My lab tests showed that the CLL was indeed progressing slowly. The doctor seemed pleased that the white cell count was stable. Apparently CLL was progressing even slower than the doctor had expected.

During 1991 and 1992 I began experiencing swelling in the lymph nodes of my neck. Eventually they got quite large, and it scared me. One, at the base of my tongue, was beginning to affect my eating and swallowing. The physician recommended a course of chemotherapy. Against my inner guidance, I agreed. I had a severe negative reaction to the chemotherapy. It was really awful.

The drugs, or maybe something else—I still don't quite know—caused a radical drop in my red blood cell count so I became extremely fatigued. I had a very strange rash and became horribly depressed. I immediately discontinued the chemotherapy but eventually had to be hospitalized for complications. Suddenly, all in just a few days, I had the frightening experience of being hospitalized, having a bone marrow biopsy, and needing to receive a blood transfusion.

I really thought I might die. My family began to send a powerful increase of prayers for me. Plus, a special drug for my kidneys helped to regenerate the red blood cell count. After a very scary experience I felt safe again. The fatigue continued for a long time, and the swelling in my neck was unchanged. A second doctor claimed that the chemotherapy dose was too large. I don't know about that, but I definitely felt poisoned.

Almost a year later I agreed to have a series of radiation treatments to try to reduce the swelling in my neck, which still was causing me difficulty when breathing and swallowing. That was scary too, but it did not cause such a horribly toxic reaction. The swelling did reduce, and I was very relieved. The doctor stated that the swelling would return in time. I was content just to feel less constrained in the neck area. That was three years ago, and my swelling has not returned.

I feel my case is a great testimony to three things that should be added to the benefits of modern medicine. First, I was amazed at how I felt immediate benefit from the increase of prayer from my family. It was very notable to me and boosted my faith. Second, I feel sure that nutrition and herbal tonics have helped me to recover my energy after the chemotherapy. Third, throughout this whole experience I have faithfully applied self-healing practices every day and felt the power of their assistance all along the way.

I believe I almost died. I wonder sometimes, "Was it just the medicine that helped me to recover?" Well, even my doctors said there is no medical therapy to improve this disorder. Yet I have had periods of what has seemed like remission. So if medicine can offer no health improvement, I must believe that the prayer and spiritual practice, the focus on nutrition, and the self-healing methods have served me very well.

Recently, I had a blood check where my white and red cell counts had returned almost to normal. Two separate doctors commented that knowing my case, they would not have expected to see such readings this many years after the diagnosis. I take that as a very positive sign.

My theory is that everything you do to heal yourself, including self-healing methods and the prayers that you send or receive, is at least as powerful as the medicine that doctors have to offer. These can work together. The healing capacity within complements and reinforces the medicine from outside. That's what they call complementary medicine, isn't it? I very definitely benefited from the radiation treatments. The chemotherapy, I still think, was a poor choice for me. My daily self-healing practice and my spiritual practice are the rock on which I have built my healing and mental calm.

Every morning I spend at least an hour doing self-healing and reading inspirational material from the Bible, and the *Daily Word*. I really believe that it is because I combine my self-healing with my practice of faith and the treatment from my doctors that I am alive today.

Margaret's Method

Over the years, the methods Margaret practices have changed from time to time. At this point it has been almost ten years since she started the practices, so she really is a kind of expert. Recently, I asked what generally caused her to make changes in her self-healing routine. She reported that every time she learned something new she would try it for a while. She keeps and uses the best techniques. Those that are less useful to her fall away. Not too long ago she borrowed some movements from Taiji and learned a new meditation. You will notice that several of her methods are ones that have stayed in her practice since she learned the self-healing methods (the same ones that are presented in this book) almost ten years ago.

> I start my practices in bed. At night as I am falling asleep I do several of the Essential Breaths and a few moments of one of the deep relaxation practices. When I awaken I use the Essential Breath again to get going. I also do what I call the "tummy rub" [similar to Massaging the Abdomen on page 72]; I've heard that it helps to reduce weight in the tummy area and it definitely helps my constipation. While still in bed I pull my knees to my chest, do the "inverted

bicycle" and the "frog." These are exercises I have invented or learned along the way. Before I go to the sitting position I do a special back exercise [the Right and Left Bending of the Spine, done lying down, page 40]. It cleared my back and hip pain so I do it faithfully.

Then I sit on the edge of the bed and do several neck stretches along with the right and left hand-to-shoulder massage and the massage of both sides of the neck with extended fingertips. I do hand and foot massage; sometimes I rub my ears too. Then I go and put water on to boil for herbal tea. While it is heating I go to my patio and do five to ten of the Front and Back Bending of the Spine and then twenty to thirty of the Flowing Motion, which has been one of my favorites. I've probably done it almost ten thousand times by now. I don't really care about living forever, so I can't imagine doing this a thousand times a day. I do like that idea of having a healthy, quality life, so I try to do one hundred a day in three or four sets. I don't imagine I've gotten to a hundred too many times, but I have already outlived the average life span for a woman so I just feel grateful.

My schedule is pretty flexible, so either after my spiritual study or later in the day I do a few of the Taiji movements that I learned recently. Other days I do the Taiji in the afternoon. Every day I try to have a walk (in nature if possible), and when I can remember, I use the In, In, Out breathing. People ask me how I can find time to do all of this. First, it doesn't really take that much time—certainly no more than any fitness program. Plus, I do it all at home so I don't spend time driving to a class or fitness center. But my most important answer is a question: would you be willing to fit a few self-healing practices into your day, or would you rather hope that the doctor can fix your cancer?

At night, in bed:

Essential Breaths (page 86)
A few moments of one of the deep relaxation practices (page 99)

In the morning, before rising:

Essential Breaths (page 86)
"Tummy rub" (similar to Massaging the Abdomen, page 72)
Several "made-up" methods
Right and Left Bending of the Spine—lying down (page 40)

Then sitting:

Right and left hand-to-shoulder massage (page 69)
Massaging the Neck (page 68)
Massaging the Hands (page 61)
Massaging the Feet (page 63)
Massaging the Ears (page 65)

Standing or moving about:

Put tea water on to boil
Front and Back Bending of the Spine (page 44)
Flowing Motion (page 37)
Cup of tea or some hot water with lemon
Study spiritual reading
Walk, in natural setting when possible
In, In, Out Breathing (page 93)
Taiji movements

The best strategy for mapping your path to self-healing or improved performance is simply to play with the methods presented in part 2. Having met with Robert, Jan, and Margaret, you can probably see that variation is desirable, safe, and inspiring. You can also draw on the tried and true routine from the Wednesday Self-Healing Practice Session in Santa Barbara (page 139).

Part 4

THE WAY OF NATURE

Nature spontaneously keeps us well. Do not resist her!

Henry David Thoreau,
transcendental philosopher and citizen activist

○

Alone, the health enhancement and self-healing methods are profound. They combine naturally with intentional focus of mind and spirit, and so the potential of the methods is multiplied. When the methods are practiced with others, their effect is amplified further still. The community of practitioners is a powerful natural force.

CHAPTER 10

Declaration of Interdependence

Unbroken wholeness denies the classical idea in science that we may analyze the world by its separate and independently existing parts.

David Bohm, physicist

YOU HAVE BECOME A KEEPER OF UNCOMMON KNOWLEDGE. You are the owner of powerful tools for health enhancement, self-healing, longevity, endurance, and vitality. You may keep and use them for the rest of your life—for free. You can give them away to others. You have studied the user's manual and have ample knowledge and inspiration to proceed with a radical upgrade in your life. Now, let us expand the domain of the practice. There is nothing additional to do. Just sustain your daily practice of the methods. The rest is automatic, the way of nature.

In their raw form and in combinations, as you have seen, the self-applied health enhancement methods are extraordinarily potent. Alone, they effectively awaken the healer within and accelerate your production of internal medicines. You may wish simply to practice for a while to explore the tools. Or you may wish to amplify the potential of your independent practice by doing the methods with others. Cultivating the influence of mind and spirit with the practice of the methods is a second powerful strategy for amplifying their potency. Both interacting purposefully with others and focusing on the interaction of mind and spirit maximize the effect of our practice through interdependence. Interdependence of body, mind, and spirit and interdependence of people within a community are expressions of a relatively new understanding in science of the interdependent nature of living systems.

The science of biology has shown that widely separated living systems are connected; they are interdependent. Small changes in a system can lead to large-scale consequences. Quantum science calls this the "butterfly effect." Because a butterfly stirring the air in Beijing could theoretically cause a storm in Seattle. Conditions in the rain forest in Brazil can have an effect on the weather and harvest in Europe.

Physiology, too, has discovered that our mental state interacts with our immune system to support or sabotage it; they, too, are interdependent. Chinese medicine is founded on the idea that our organ systems and emotions cooperate interdependently in health. Disease can exist only if the harmonious interaction of the organs and emotions is malfunctioning. Physics has found that all forms in the universe spring from a single origin. Each particular event or thing is woven into the unified whole.

The wisdom teachings of the world's great spiritual traditions agree. They declare that all of the various phenomena in the universe are contained within the singular, divine body of God. Both scientific and spiritual traditions put forth the idea that all things and forces are in a powerful and dynamic relationship. When we each take on the responsibility to sustain the health of our own little piece of the universe, then we are cooperating to sustain the health of the whole.

The whole what? you ask. Well, the whole self, the whole family, the whole culture, and even the whole world. For example, the earth is an independent celestial body. Yet it is impossible to imagine what the earth would be without its relationship with the sun, moon, and other planets in our solar system. I am a wildly independent individual, but I would be far less whole without my family, friends, and professional alliances. Interdependence makes independence more potent, more fun.

Just as our body is worth caring for because it is the dwelling place of our self, the world is worth caring for because it is the dwelling place of our selves. But becoming interdependent sounds like an immense project, kind of like trying to save the world. Don't waste good energy being overwhelmed. The beauty of the nature of living systems is that you support the potential of the whole simply by doing your own part. Without leaving your own home, you are collaborating interdependently with all other participants in this healing revolution. Take just a moment to understand this deeply. By simply doing your own practice you are a participant in something positive, something grand.

Solo Practice: Independence

Doing health enhancement practices is a little like taking a first step toward fully self-directed living. Remember how your first two-wheel bike had training wheels? The health enhancement methods are like self-reliance training wheels.

The location for your practice, the length of your practice period, the part of the day when you practice, and the specific methods you explore are all up to you when you practice alone. You don't have to wait for anyone, convince anyone, or accommodate anyone. One day you may practice for a short period, the next day you may practice for a long time. Maybe you only want to meditate today and skip the other practices. Perhaps a big holiday is coming and you need extra energy; you can expand your practice for a few days to build up your endurance. Or you may be preparing for a sports event, so you can modify your practice to complement your training.

By activating the healer within, an individual becomes stronger and healthier without having to take on a large project or focus. Even a tiny bit of practice can be a huge advance in the right direction. When broken down into small, attainable steps, a health enhancement practice can help an individual to build the energy and confidence necessary to take on larger projects in life.

The loss of a job or a loved one can be paralyzing. Elizabeth, whom we met in chapter 1, lost her husband, her motivation, and her health all at once. This is not an unusual sequence of events. Recall that she rebounded very positively both physically and emotionally when she began to practice gentle self-healing methods.

She went from crawling to the bathroom to a trip to Alaska. Using the self-applied health enhancement methods helps a person to regain and reactivate his or her own inner strength.

With a challenging disease like cancer or multiple sclerosis, it is only possible to spend a few moments with the doctor on an occasional basis, perhaps every two to four weeks. Yet to heal genuinely, one needs to implement health enhancement choices and activities frequently, throughout every day. People often believe that the physician or the drug or the surgical procedure is the focus of their approach to a health problem; they fail to recognize the importance of the healer within. Through the self-healing practices, individuals can accelerate their healing every day, even several times a day, completely on their own if they wish.

Find the best room in your house for your practice and arrange the furnishings, modify the light, and perhaps allow for music. Notice that it is particularly pleasant to practice outdoors where nature's healing resources are particularly potent. Solo practice allows you to choose your own favorite practice spot. See if you can tell the difference when you practice near trees, by water, or in the mountains. When you practice by yourself you are alone with the healer within and with the powerful healing forces of nature.

Helping Yourself Helps Everyone

When you use these practices to enhance yourself, or heal yourself, it helps others in a number of ways. Your personal health will improve. This will reduce the cost of health care in your family. It will make you more available to others and make it more fun to be around you. Those who are well always experience greater productivity and clearer decision making than those who are sick. No one would deny that feeling well enhances creativity, joy, and the ability to act with vitality.

When you help yourself in this way, you are liberated from your dependence on others, and they are freed from your dependence on them. At the same time the power of personal independence strengthens the family and the community. When a group of independent individuals interacts, it is not dependence or codependence. It is cooperative interdependence. A group of self-sufficient and independent citizens can cooperate to produce a greater outcome than can be achieved by a group in which some participants are self-reliant and others are not.

This is the premise behind the old-fashioned "barn raising." A group of self-reliant, capable neighbors would get together to build a barn, something that one self-reliant individual could not accomplish alone. This ability of capable individuals to work together is an expression of the best definition of community. It is this quality of community—spirited interdependence—that revolutionary nations (the United States, France, and others) celebrate as they look back at their own history.

In earlier times self-reliant individuals cooperated interdependently to harvest their crops, protect their communities, and even redefine their nations. Today the challenges have changed. Now we cooperate as capable individuals to protect the air and water, strengthen families, eliminate violence and war, and reduce the waste of financial and natural resources. Each healthy, self-reliant citizen can play his or her part in solving larger challenges by effectively caring for himself or herself.

The self-applied health enhancement methods are useful tools with which to reach for self-empowerment and personal freedom. They can help to reduce the costs associated with illness. They are also tools that we can use to strengthen our communities. They can help to provide a foundation for an individual's personal welfare. Each independent person who individually takes action to enhance his or her health strengthens the interdependent whole.

Transforming Health Care for a New Century

Nearly one trillion dollars is spent on health care and medicine in the United States in one year. Using the official estimate of the Department of Health and Human Services that 70 percent of all diseases are preventable, estimate the possibilities. When we work together to increase our health, an immense economic return becomes available. In very simple terms we could say that 70 percent of a trillion dollars could be saved and used differently. Earlier we figured in a certain expense for prevention, so approximately five hundred billion dollars could be saved.

Just imagine a scenario in which every able individual began to practice the health-enhancing and self-healing methods we have been exploring here. Clearly the methods are easy enough to learn. Obviously they are easy to practice. There is no cost for their application. They can even be passed among friends or from elders to children. The practical barriers to the widespread use of these ideas and practices are minimum.

Imagine every able individual is taking care of himself or herself. The 70 percent of diseases and injuries that are potentially preventable have been prevented. The five hundred billion dollars of clinical and administrative health care expenses have been saved. What would you choose, as a representative of your community, to spend those dollars on? In my conversations with people all over North America I have had many responses to this question. A few of the answers include: eliminating crime, returning art and music to our schools, developing technologies for building houses and packaging products without destroying forests, paying off the national debt, maximizing reusable resources, upgrading bridges and roads, and helping developing countries skip the phase of development where pollution from leaded fuel and high-sulfur coal is uncontrolled. What would you choose?

When you begin to use these self-healing practices, you may also begin to consider how you would spend the health care dollars that you are responsible for saving. After all, they are *your* dollars. When we do not take responsibility for our health, we have little right to question how health care dollars are spent. But when we are vigilant in making choices and taking actions that sustain health, then it becomes our right and responsibility to redirect the dollars that we save.

Practicing with Others: Interdependence

At a training in New York a man commented after a period of group practice, "That was one of my best meditations. Why do I seem to have deeper meditations when I practice with others?" In

1995 I was invited by the Institute of Noetic Sciences to lead the audience in a group activity, drawing on the self-healing and health enhancement methods. There were approximately 1,500 people present. Immediately preceding the keynote presentation we spent fifteen minutes practicing together. Afterward dozens of people stopped me to say, "In that brief practice with the group, I experienced something unusual, something that I don't often feel in my own practice!"

It is typical for people to have a sense of gaining more or accomplishing more when they interact with a group. Whether it is a work group, a support group, a study group, a worship group, or a group devoted to the self-healing arts, people tend to accomplish more in a concerted group process.

Nearly a thousand people have made over ten thousand visits to our Wednesday Self-Healing Practice Session during the six-year period of its existence. Each of them brought their own unique expression to the practices. Frequently, they would share exciting testimonies of the benefits they were experiencing. Many of them came several times, learned the practices, and then continued the application on their own. Some were visiting from homes in other parts of the country and even around the world.

Many others were regular attendees. While all of them reported the value of their solo practice, many also mentioned their fondness for the group practice session. It became necessary at one point to put the group practice on hold during a period when I was going to be traveling. During that period the Health Action Clinic received frequent calls from the "regulars" stating that they missed the group practice. Some reported that the group session helped them to keep their personal practice going; in other words, the interdependence fostered independence. Some reported that the group practice helped them to reach a deeper state of relaxation. Others felt that the weekly meeting was their favorite social time because the participants were all like-minded and enthusiastic. The desire to practice with a group led to the creation of additional meeting sites and times, led by various members. For example, several began to meet on Fridays to practice together, using videos. Another group began to meet in a park on Sundays.

Experiencing Chinese Group Practice

Following their group practice of the self-healing methods, the members of the Cancer Recovery Society, whom we first met in chapter 6, also practice what is called "social oncology." Oncology is the study of cancer; a physician whose special area of expertise is cancer is called an oncologist. What, then, is social oncology?

During a visit to China in 1991, I got the answer to this question, and it revealed to me the profound healing possibilities that are often overlooked in our conventional system of medicine as well as in our social sciences. Social oncology is human interaction with the purpose of supporting the recovery of health by people with cancer. Social immunology and social cardiology would be human interaction to support the recovery of the immune and cardiac functions.

My most cherished clinical experiences with Chinese medicine had revealed to me that the true healer lies within and that each person produces his or her own medicines internally. What had not become fully obvious until that visit to China is that we can help activate this medicine in each other. Meeting with the Cancer Recovery Society gave me one of the most potent demonstrations of the healing value of human interaction that I had ever witnessed.

The cancer recovery groups meet to practice their self-healing methods in the parks throughout China, particularly in Beijing and Shanghai. They practice Guo Lin's Cancer Recovery Qigong (Chi Kung), which is named for the woman who developed the methods in the 1960s. She adapted a self-healing form that she had learned from her grandfather. After the practice the group gathers in a nearby teahouse to drink Chinese green tea and socialize. Many of China's parks have lovely teahouses. And scientific research in herbal medicine has found that green tea has immune-enhancing properties.

For about an hour the group then engages in social oncology. This includes the singing of lighthearted songs, the telling of jokes, lots of laughter, lighthearted philosophical discussion and debate, the introduction of new members, the reading of poems and stories that highlight the possibilities of recovery from cancer, reminders that cancer does not necessarily equal death, and the sharing of inspiring personal cancer recovery testimonials.

As a part of the gathering the group sings "Happy Birthday" in Chinese (and in English, perhaps because of my presence) to each person for whom the day is the anniversary of their cancer diagnosis. I was particularly astounded on my first visit with the Cancer Recovery Society to be present for an elder gentleman's thirtieth anniversary of his diagnosis of cancer. Several years later I witnessed one of the cancer recovery groups celebrating a woman's fifth year of recovery since her diagnosis of liver cancer. The conventionally recognized survival period for liver cancer is under three years. She was looking radiantly healthy at five years.

I have asked dozens of members of the Cancer Recovery Society for their opinion on the value of "social oncology." Their responses have fallen into three categories. The first speaks of its power to reduce stress and is captured in this statement by Zao Ling Xiu: "The social healing part of our recovery program serves as a constant reminder that healing is enhanced when we are light of heart and free of worry."

Zhou Pei expresses the second value of the social interaction, the power of testimony: "We do not need much scientific evidence to prove the value of our cancer recovery program; each day in our social healing session we hear the stories of our close recovery friends who prove that we can save ourselves from sickness and death." The third, the value of love and encouragement from friends, is best stated by Yuan Zheng Ping, the director of the Shanghai Cancer Recovery Society, who said, "Depression and fear, worry and isolation are like food to cancer. Social oncology provides fun, deep caring connection, encouragement, and inspiration, which are the enemies of disease. Recovery is significantly enhanced by the social aspect of our program."

At a lovely Chinese banquet in 1995, I was honored to meet with the minister of public health of one of China's most ancient and famous cities, Hangzhou. I asked if the morning practice of self-healing in the parks is considered to be an official public health program. "In China we have a very strong social vision," he said. "It is a primary feature of our traditional system of medicine to sustain a high level of health in our large population," which numbers over a billion people. "Our primary prevention strategy is to support the practice of Chinese health enhancement and self-healing, which people carry out in their homes and in the public parks. While this is largely a social activity, it has very favorable medical results. Many of the teachers in the parks are retired doctors, teachers, and politicians. It is a part of our social vision to honor and revere the wisdom of the elders. These citizens accept the cultural responsibility to pass health knowledge down to younger generations. The cost of these programs is very, very small. The Chinese people have been interested in health and longevity for thousands of years. This is an official program, but it happens with no effort; it is automatic."

Finding Like-Minded Friends

Emphasizing the benefits of group practice is not intended to overshadow the value of personal practice. Allow your solo practice to be the heart of your daily health enhancement activity. If it seems right, seek like-minded friends to practice with and share experiences. In China, this is easy. In Santa Barbara, where I live, little self-healing groups have begun to spring up here and there.

I have lectured all over the United States and Canada as well as in China and Puerto Rico and have found that interested and enthusiastic people are always in abundant supply. If you want to practice with a group, I guarantee you can find others who share your interest.

In 1984 I was hired by a major district medical center in Aibonito, Puerto Rico, to help them establish an acupuncture program in their community clinic and develop a community wellness program. I led a class in the self-applied health enhancement methods on several mornings at the hospital's community outpatient clinic and found many self-care friends. There were usually from fifty to seventy-five people in the waiting room who participated. Everyone laughed as I tried out my minimal Spanish. Children were skipping and singing among the group. At one point a patient brought a small pig in a burlap bag as extra payment for his doctor, and the pig was squealing as he walked through the waiting room. No one noticed; we just kept rubbing our ears and doing our deep breathing practices.

On my last trip to China I led a group of twenty-five people who wanted to study Chinese Qigong self-healing. We were traveling in the spectacular Huang Mountains when we became aware that another group of self-healing enthusiasts, thirty people from Fukuoka, Japan, were staying in the same hotel high in the mountains. They called themselves the Fukuoka Qigong Family, and they had come, like us, to practice Qigong in the rarefied energy of ancient, revered mountains.

A coincidence? Not really. On other trips to China I have met groups from Germany, France, Sweden, Australia, Japan, and America who were studying Qigong. No matter where you are, others with this same interest are not far away. Call the phone number or connect with the Internet address on pages 257–258, and we will help you find a group nearby or suggest how you might gather some people together in your community (see also the appendix).

As your practice continues, you will begin to run into people in your community who are interested in health enhancement or who have been inspired by this book. Most YMCAs have daily low-impact exercise classes that are consistent with these self-healing concepts. Watch the schedule of your local continuing education or community recreation institutions for self-healing classes, including the self-applied health enhancement methods (SAHEM), Yoga, Qigong, Taiji (Tai Chi), low-impact aerobics, meditation, acupressure, and massage. Most hospitals have begun to sponsor such programs as well.

Several sites on the Internet will assist you in finding health enhancement friends; many libraries and health centers have computers that access the Internet. Television links to the Internet are also available. Search for "self-healing, "health enhancement," "Qigong," "Chi Kung," "Taiji," and "Yoga." Two sites that have excellent self-healing information are healthworld.com and wellness.com. Look for "directories" where you can link with people in your area, find information on practice sessions, and locate instructors. Look for "libraries" where you can find information to enrich your health enhancement knowledge base. Look for "practices" where you can learn new self-healing methods. Look for "forums" where you can actually carry on conversations with self-healing and self-care friends from all over the world.

The self-healing revolution is dramatically accelerated when the value of interdependence is embraced. This is why groups practice together in China; social interaction has a healing effect, as the Cancer Recovery Society has shown. Group-based support and study are some of the most powerful aspects of the emerging new health care system, which we will explore in more detail in the next chapters. And as you will find in part 5, the Chinese have discovered some even more promising effects of group practice that will dramatically alter our understanding of interdependence.

CHAPTER 11

The Empowering Influence of Mind and Spirit

The greatest revolution of our generation is the discovery that human beings, by changing the inner attitudes of their minds, can change the outer aspects of their lives.

William James,
psychologist, philosopher

ON THE FIRST PAGES OF THIS BOOK YOU MET PATRICIA, who spontaneously discovered her own capacity for self-healing. She combined breath practice and deep relaxation with faith and saved her own life. To the surprise of her physician team, who predicted that they might have to remove her spleen to save her, she walked away from an emergency situation needing neither surgery nor medication. Patricia felt that her faith was a key component of her self-healing experience.

By combining the self-applied health enhancement methods with purposeful attention to mind and spirit we can awaken the greatest response of the healer within. The self-healing methods alone are powerful. With the added influence of mind and spirit, the methods are maximized.

Influence—the word itself is a teacher. It means "an intangible force that affects the flow of circumstances" or "to change the course of events." *Influence* is such a commonly used word that we miss its true meaning, which points to a power that affects the flow of our experiences. The flow of health and vitality is affected significantly by thoughts, feelings, and beliefs. Although these are generally thought of as being related to mind alone, the biological activity associated with these influences is significant. "Mind-body medicine," "attitudinal healing," "behavioral medicine," and "psychoneuroimmunology" are some of the phrases used in health care to describe the influence of mind and spirit on health. Attitudes and emotions have always been explored by scientists and philosophers. The mind and even faith have now been scrutinized under the light of science.

The Heroes of Mind-Body Interaction

Hippocrates, the father of Western medicine, taught doctors to gain their patients' faith and observe their life circumstances and emotional states. Socrates agreed, declaring, "Curing the soul; that is the first thing."

The Judeo-Christian tradition speaks to attitudes and emotions repeatedly: "a cheerful heart is good medicine, but a crushed spirit dries up the bones," and "your faith has healed you, go in peace." The ancient Chinese medical system has at its foundation several guidelines that indicate the importance of mind and spirit. The first rule of the physician of traditional Chinese medicine is "Honor the spirit."

In the final moments of the twentieth century a virtual landslide of scientific evidence has confirmed the powerful influence of mind and spirit in healing. Numerous excellent books have translated this immense body of information into exciting and useful fuel for the self-healing revolution. Writers such as Dean Ornish, Larry Dossey, Christiane Northrup, Joan Borysenko, Bernie Siegel, Norman Shealy, Andrew Weil, Deepak Chopra, David Eisenburg, and Herbert Benson are the pioneering voices in a profound discussion about holistic medicine, self-healing, and the healing influences of mind and spirit. And they stand on the shoulders of Walter Cannon, probably the first modern scientist who made the body-mind connection decades earlier, and Hans Selye, who detailed the physiological impact of stress on the body and stated emphatically that the body produces both dangerous poisons and marvelous medicines. (These authors' books are noted under "Bibliography and Suggested Reading," page 249.) We can now see the marvel of self-healing and health enhancement because we are standing on the shoulders of these giants and their ancient ancestors from China, India, and other original cultures.

Norman Cousins, former editor of the *Saturday Review*, became one of the most notable spokespersons for the power of mind and spirit in self-healing when he recovered from an incurable collagen disorder in part through de-stressing his system by watching humorous films. In a number of excellent books he brilliantly clarified the power of self-healing. This quotation from *Human Options* eloquently captures the essence of my message about the healer within:

> Over the years, medical science has identified the primary systems of the human body: the circulatory system, digestive system, endocrine system, autonomic nervous system and the immune system. But two other systems that are central to the proper functioning of a human being need to be emphasized. The healing system and the belief system. The two work together. (Cousins, 1981)

When we trigger the healing system with the self-applied health enhancement methods and then also trigger the power of the belief system, the capacity for heightened human potential and for recovery from disease is greatly magnified. From ancient times through the present, the most revered healers have known that the human being has a vital self-healing capacity that is profoundly influenced by faith and emotional harmony. We are entering an era where this understanding of self-healing will become as common as aspirin and antibiotics have been in the recent past.

The Influences: Emotions, Belief, Humor

To understand the influence of mind and spirit on self-healing, we will explore briefly in the sections that follow a number of related areas. *Emotions* have now been thoroughly explored by science. The effect of *humor* in healing is well documented. Excellent research on placebos, remissions, and miracles reflects the healing influence of *belief*. *Faith*, both sacred and practical, has also received scientific attention. The research regarding *forgiveness* and *surrender* is less complete, but these are powerful mental and spiritual factors in self-healing, as you will see. We will also explore how *group support, accountability,* and *testimonials* foster the ability of individuals to embrace and work with mind and spirit influences.

Emotions

The scientific research on the effect of emotions on health can be stated simply. Body chemistry shifts and literally produces poisons when a person is in a sustained state of anger, fear, grief, frustration, or worry. Physiologically, when a person is in a stress state, the overactivity of the nervous system taxes the adrenal gland. This creates a lack of responsiveness in the body's self-healing capacity. The immune cells are unable to get clear direction when the adrenal is overactive or deficient, leading to risk of cancer and other immune deficiency disorders. And stress builds tension in the circulatory system, elevating the risk of heart attack or stroke.

These findings have been reconfirmed in hundreds of studies. It has also been clearly established that sustained joy, contentment, and security cause a shift in the body chemistry to produce healing elixirs. In a classic study, scientists at the Clinical Neuroendocrinological Laboratory at the National Institutes of Health in Washington, D.C., found that patients with depression are in a state of chronic low-grade anxiety, secreting high quantities of the body chemicals associated with stress (Gold, 1987). In a collaborative study at Stanford and Emory Universities, researchers found that depressed individuals sustained high levels of stress hormones in their blood. They showed depleted energy reserves and suppressed immune function.

The self-healing methods turn on the inner medicines that can neutralize negative emotional influences. When support and social interaction help to trigger the positive influences of laughter, communication, and sharing, health improves. When hate is transformed by joy, the heart is healed. When worry is transformed by calm, the immune function is boosted. Notice that moving the body, deepening the breath, and doing a little self-massage can also shift your mood.

Belief

Centuries ago, belief—sometimes referred to as superstition—was a significant aspect of healing. As science developed, it became clear that ancient doctors would sometimes use methods that were effective precisely because they triggered the patient's beliefs. A classic example of this is a story told by medical anthropologists. A doctor in Africa who was dealing with a woman who had terrible stomach discomfort used a particularly obvious, quite effective, and somewhat devious cure. He announced that her sickness was caused by an evil creature that had entered her body. Then he gave her an herbal formula that he promised would heal the stomach problem. It was actually an emetic formula that almost immediately caused violent vomiting. Soon the patient was retching so vigorously that her eyes were watering profusely and were forced shut. While she was engaged in the vomiting spree, the doctor removed a small pet snake from a container among his medicine tools, and he placed the snake in the bowl that she was vomiting into. He began exclaiming that she was cured. When she was able to open her eyes, she saw the snake and was amazed. From then on her stomach improved, which she attributed to the doctor's brilliant choice of herbs and astute diagnostic skills.

In this case the doctor clearly healed the patient by drawing on the power of belief. Because the use of belief in medicine has sometimes been associated with deception, it has also become associated with the abuse of people's genuine desire to be healed. With the advent of the modern scientific era, medicine that was based on influences that engaged the mind—belief, emotional states, and attitudes—became associated with unscientific ideas and superstitions. The ancient doctors who used these tools were considered by "sophisticated" Western scientists to be primitive and uneducated. In more recent times doctors and healers who have used such methods have been called quacks and charlatans.

But the role of belief in healing has now been redeemed by science. The new holistic approach to medicine and healing supports belief in both the "art" of healing and the "science" of medicine. You can believe in God, science, energies, angels, technology, herbs, or surgery—it doesn't matter what you believe in; the healing influence of belief causes the body to produce the same internal chemicals in all cases. Belief amplifies the effects of your self-healing practice. And because you will experience a positive benefit from practice, your practice will amplify your belief.

Humor

Humor and lightheartedness are tremendous healers. Norman Cousins's case exemplified this so dramatically that he was invited to take a post at the prestigious UCLA Medical School. His book *Head First: The Biology of Hope* is the story of helping physicians to break through their professional and academic barriers to the
+ mind-body interaction. The science of psychoneuroimmunology (PNI) has found that when laughter occurs, the body produces healing chemicals that enhance immune function and reduce pain.

The medical literature has dozens of citings of the impact of humor on health. Studies in the *American Journal of Medical Science* revealed that when people laughed the body decreased production of stress hormones and increased production of the inner medicines (Berk, 1989). The *Journal of the Academy of Nurse Practitioners* published a study that identified humor as a key skill in the delivery of health care services (Lewis, 1994). The *Journal of Heart and Lung Transplant* found that the top two strategies for patients coping with the wait for an organ transplant were positive thinking and humor (Grady, 1995). And it was reported in the journal *Cancer Nurse* that humor has a genuine therapeutic effect (Bellert, 1989).

When you bring humor to your daily practice of the self-healing methods, it multiplies the benefit. One morning in

Hangzhou, China, I watched a man doing his self-healing practices facing a large tree. For about three to four minutes he would wiggle and bounce his body about, as in the Spontaneous Movement (page 51). At times he added self-massage, rubbing his shoulders and working on his neck (page 68). Next he would do a movement similar to the Gathering Breath (page 96), and then he would become very still for a moment. Suddenly, he would break out in hilarious laughter for twelve to fifteen seconds. Finally, he would stand quietly for a few moments and then start the whole process again. I walked away after three or four rounds, but he just kept on going.

It is not unusual for our Wednesday morning practice group to have a good laugh. Someone makes a silly comment or sings a few lines from a song that fits the moment, and everybody laughs. "I love it when we laugh," people say. The Cancer Recovery Society in Shanghai makes laughter a top priority in its "social oncology." During several of my visits, when a good laugh arose, the director would turn to me and smile. Through the interpreter he said, "This is our strongest medicine."

The Sacred: Faith, Forgiveness, and Surrender

Many people find that their practice of self-healing methods feels sacred. Both Jan and Margaret, whom we met earlier, associate their self-healing methods with their spiritual practice. In November 1994, *Newsweek* reported that 45 percent of people who meditate feel a sense of the sacred. Earlier the same year a Gallup poll found that 90 percent of Americans pray, feel that their prayers are answered, and are mindful of health and well-being in their prayers.

Faith

Faith has received a fair amount of attention from science. Dr. Herbert Benson from the Harvard Medical School has nicely explored faith in healing in his most recent book, *Timeless Healing*. He borrows the term *faith factor* from a fascinating volume published by the John Templeton Foundation, *The Faith Factor: An Annotated Bibliography of Clinical Research on Spiritual Subjects*

(Mathews, 1993). The writers found that religious factors assisted in several health areas: reduced use of alcohol, cigarettes, and drugs; reduced anxiety, depression, and anger; reduced blood pressure; and improved quality of life for patients with cancer and heart disease. In fifteen out of sixteen studies that they explored, exposure to religious activities generated greater well-being. In 100 percent of the studies they reviewed, they found that exposure to religious activities reduced hostility. In 100 percent of the studies, they found reduced cigarette and drug use. At Eastern Virginia University Medical School doctors found by reviewing hundreds of research articles that faith in God lowers premature death rates and enhances health (Levin, 1994).

Specific examples of the "faith factor" include a study at Northwestern University where elderly women with strong religious beliefs who were recovering from hip correction surgeries were able to walk significantly longer distances than those without such beliefs (Pressman, 1990). At Dartmouth Medical School it was found that heart disease patients who received solace and comfort from their religious faith were three times more likely to survive than those who did not (Oxman, 1995).

When you bring the benefits of faith to your practice of the health enhancement and self-healing methods, the potential benefits are doubled. Presentations on the health enhancement methods and the PHASES program have been especially interesting in hospitals with religious affiliations and with health ministry and parish nurse programs because the "faith factor" is prevalent.

Forgiveness and Surrender

The light of science, I feel sure, will one day confirm the healing power of forgiveness and surrender (acceptance). They are part of the art of healing but not yet a part of the science of medicine. I mention them here because there is a tremendous tension in holding a grudge and fighting against the natural flow of events. Ancient traditional systems of medicine believed that holding a grudge and fighting against the natural flow of events drain vitality. One of my patients who was challenged with cancer is a poignant example of this. She was completely conscious of how her unhappy relationship with her husband was sabotaging her ability to heal. She declared, "I cannot forgive my husband, and it is killing me."

Similarly, the inability to surrender to or accept that which is obviously meant to be drains vitality. In the most refined systems of self-healing, the ability to forgive and the ability to accept certain inevitable events are considered the greatest healers. In some forms of Qigong (Chi Kung) from China and of Yoga from India, the capacities to forgive and surrender are the most elevated forms of healing and are called soul healing. These systems propose that when the soul is healed, it automatically clears the mind, and this automatically heals the body. When one forgives, a certain injurious tension is released. When one accepts the unfolding of life with its many heartbreaks, disappointments, and victories, one is liberated from a dangerous inner strain. During your practice, in that quiet that you will find, explore the possibilities of forgiveness and surrender. Notice that it is not the unforgiven person who suffers but the unforgiving one. Notice also that surrender liberates you from trying to change what cannot be changed.

Methods for Mobilizing the Influence of Mind and Spirit

There are resources that foster balanced emotions, empowered belief systems, and the exposure to the sacred. These include solid families with wise elders who pass down traditional knowledge, as well as harmonious communities where everyone helps each other to get along. In a dream community, churches, schools, businesses, hospitals, and even jails would cooperate in this. We, however, live in high-pressure, changing times. Even intact families are extremely busy, while communities comprise numerous layers of economic and social complexity. As a result, stress is high, emotions are strained, and belief systems are insecure.

There are methods that help to neutralize negative emotions and self-sabotaging beliefs and that favor humor and nurture faith, forgiveness, and surrender in people's lives. These tools—group support, accountability, and testimonials—are potent resources that can help rebuild families and bring harmony to communities.

Group or Team Support

Interaction with others can help people transform their attitudes and emotions. This magnifies the effect of the self-healing and health enhancement methods. Health care providers and businesses have found that focused interaction among people can increase health and productivity. Support-group activity in health care and teamwork in business set in motion emotional and attitudinal changes.

Until recently, our culture fostered an overreliance on experts in medicine, education, and business. Access to healing required a medical expert. Learning depended on a teacher. Success in business depended on the expertise of the boss, manager, or supervisor. Fortunately, a dramatic transformation is occurring in many professions. In order to reduce expenses and improve productivity and profit, businesses are eliminating experts (managers) and giving more power and responsibility to employees. Health care organizations, to reduce expenses and improve health, are giving more power and responsibility to the patients or clients themselves. In both cases the dynamic interaction among people is a powerful key to improved results. In business this interaction takes place primarily within the "self-directed team." In education "learning teams" have become common. In health care a powerful new focus of interaction is the "peer support group" or "health improvement team." These groups have the same design as that of the Cancer Recovery Society in China: group support and study are combined with self-healing methods.

With both teams and group support or group study, the participants become experts for each other. Because information on so many topics is now readily accessible (in books and through the Internet, for instance), participants can frequently inform each other in situations that formerly would have required an expert. The expert does not disappear but instead is used more prudently. A powerful new dynamic emerges from this change. If you enable individuals to be self-reliant and then encourage self-reliant individuals to interact, problems will be resolved.

The keys are support, accountability, and communication. Take a moment to explore this. First, get a feel for this phrase: "I hope I can find an expert who can heal me." Now get a feel for this phrase: "I will activate the natural healing resources within me to help heal myself." In one you are passive. In the other you are active. They are not exclusive; both can operate simultaneously.

In 1983 at the Health Action Clinic, we were redesigning our health care delivery to focus on health rather than disease. We discovered right away that customers need access to information and interaction with each other. We originally thought that classes led by experts were the best way to deliver that information. Quickly it became obvious that this was far less powerful and a whole lot more costly than allowing participants to inform each other. The original classes were set up with the lecturing expert addressing a group of people who sat in rows facing him or her. We found pretty quickly that it was better to put the chairs in a circle and have the expert facilitate a more interactive process of learning and support. The circle discussion was moderated by the facilitator, but the substance of the discussion, in terms of both support and information, came from the participants. Finally, in some cases the facilitator was removed and the group became self-directed. This evolved into the PHASES program, a process that assists people in improving their health and performance in phases or steps (see the appendix, page 246).

Participants in PHASES were able to help each other improve their health with little expert input. It was humbling and exciting for me, an expert myself. In the support and study groups, communication and trust became the primary focus, even more so than information exchange. An entirely different way of dealing with people who were sick was emerging, based on information, learning, social interaction, individual action, support, and accountability. Acupuncture, herbal medicine, homeopathy, and massage became secondary to group activities, either support and learning groups or health improvement teams.

By 1988 or so, we were hosting numerous support and study groups for cancer, AIDS, and chronic fatigue syndrome using the PHASES model. We were also using PHASES in corporate health promotion programs. Both medical and business literature began to report studies that confirmed the value of social support for patients and employees. Early research on the benefits of social interaction at the University of Michigan, the University of Texas, Stanford, and Yale found that participants who experienced social interaction were two to three times less likely to die from their diagnosed disease than those who were isolated (Berkman, 1979). Married cancer patients did better medically than those who were unmarried (Goodwin, 1987). In an interesting study at Stanford that is somewhat distressing to animal lovers like myself, monkeys were put under the stress of receiving repeated electrical shocks. When the monkey was alone, the stress was radically debilitating. However, with as few as five "friends" present, the negative effect of the shocks was completely neutralized (Levine, 1989).

Probably the most often cited study of the effect of support was conducted in a randomized clinical trial by Dr. David Spiegel at Stanford with eighty-six women with metastatic breast cancer (Spiegel, 1989). The study was originally intended to explore the effect of support on levels of anxiety, depression, fatigue, and mood disturbance. It was found that the fifty women in the support groups did significantly better than the thirty-six women who received regular cancer treatment without participating in the groups.

Dr. Spiegel was surprised to find, on further analysis of the data, that the women in the support groups also had a substantial extension of the length of their lives. He had originally doubted that the support group would affect longevity, so the original focus of the support activity was not to lengthen life but only to improve the quality of life. This study and others like it have confirmed the idea that group interaction can enhance quality and even length of life in cases of serious health challenge. In business the concept of teamwork has been found to greatly enhance productivity, communication, and conflict resolution skills.

Along with the health enhancement methods, group interaction is probably one of the breakthrough features of health care delivery for the twenty-first century. At Health Action we have evaluated the impressions of participants in numerous groups (support, study, practice) over the years and compiled a list of benefits of team interaction or group activity. Most often, in these groups, the health enhancement and self-healing methods were combined with the PHASES program in what we call "a process of continuous personal improvement." Whether at the clinic or in hospitals, schools, or businesses, people reported pretty much the same benefits from group interaction. Those most frequently reported include

> Provides access to knowledge
> Increases feelings of empowerment
> Offers a sense of partnership
> Feels like a family
> Helps with coping
> Makes you feel less like a victim
> Creates a sense of community and safety
> Offers a safe environment where you can release tension and express feelings
> Provides inspiration through the stories of others (testimonials)
> Offers more learning through other participants than you can get from a doctor or boss
> Builds trust
> Encourages a cooperative approach to problem solving
> Fosters clear communication
> Helps to change behaviors and thoughts
> Increases self-esteem
> Supports taking control and self-reliance
> Leads to personal insight
> Offers connection and sharing with others
> Provides an energy exchange
> Produces a more holistic process
> Encourages personal action
> Requires accountability
> Improves health or productivity through learning and communication

Accountability

Accountability is an important feature of support, and it is essential to self-reliance and your health enhancement practice. Whether in health care or in business, once the focus has shifted to include personal improvement or team activity, accountability becomes fundamental. What is accountability? It sounds so removed from the language of self-healing. Simply stated, accountability is the willingness to take responsibility for one's actions. To be accountable is to be true to one's word.

To be accountable for honesty, purposeful work, joyfulness, service, family time, and play is one of your most potent tools for improvement of health or personal performance, because it means that you do what you say you will do. Accountability is identical to integrity. Accountability in your self-healing practice is actually doing the practice.

In the context of healing or in enhancing performance in business, the goal is improvement—improved health or improved productivity and profitability. Success is dependent on accountability in both fields. At Health Action we have explored the support and health enhancement process over and over to see if we could discover the richest, most essential feature of supportive interaction or personal improvement. Accountability is the essence. It is the ability to honor the goals you have set. In all of the areas of choice that we have discussed—attitude, lifestyle, and self-care—your results will be spectacular when accountability is present. Without accountability your choices in these areas are meaningless.

So many times I have heard people with dangerous diseases say, "This disease has given me a gift," or "This disease is the most important thing that has ever happened to me." Such statements have always puzzled me. I try to imagine—if I had severe cancer or AIDS, could I say it was a gift?

Rebecca, my favorite colleague and also my wife, who has been facilitating healing support and study groups, individual transformation, and corporate teams for years, explains it like this: "When people reach the point where they are no longer willing to be victims, when they become accountable for the quality of their experience, they are reborn, transformed. At that point it doesn't matter so much if they have this job or that job. It doesn't matter so much whether their life is brief or lengthy. The quality of their life is radically improved. Guilt, worry, and uncontrollable fear have been cast out. Joy and trust can be purposefully invited to enter their lives. It doesn't matter so much what is happening. How they react to what is happening becomes the focus, and the richness of their life expands. Accountable for the nature of their experience, they can elect to banish frustration, fear, and the torment of continuous stress. They enter a new life where they literally radiate, and enthusiasm can flourish."

Those who master accountability are literally reborn through their own labor. Biologically this rebirth produces a fantastic medicine within the human system. Together with the health enhancement and self-healing methods, accountability is an astounding force. Accountability in relation to the self-healing methods produces vigilant practice, and vigilant practice makes miracles possible.

Testimonials

Another unusual feature that dramatically supports personal change is the surprising power of the testimonial. In medical science, the testimonial, also known as anecdotal evidence, is considered useless as proof of the benefit or value of a medical treatment. In former eras, testimonials and anecdotes were used by unscrupulous salespeople who were selling unproved medicines that often contained alcohol or opium. The Food and Drug Administration (FDA) was created to protect consumers from medicines that were dangerous or had no value. Similarly, the American Medical Association was formed, in part, to protect people from unscrupulous salespeople making dishonest medical claims.

In protecting people from the dark side of the testimonial, these agencies have also made it more difficult to benefit from the healing power of people's stories of recovery. But we are in a new era. We can now carefully draw on the benefit of testimonials, even while we continue to protect people from dishonesty. The body of rigorous scientific literature on the power of the testimonial is small but growing.

What we have found empirically, through working with individuals and groups, is that there is a resident wisdom within each person. When an individual begins to polish the dust and dirt off his or her essential nature, that wisdom can radiate through. When incorrect information, reactive emotions, and false attitudes that spring from fear and guilt are polished away, the light of wisdom shines. Because personal wisdom has been distrusted during the era when only experts had authority, the value of the testimonial, of one individual's story, has seemed insignificant. However, when people work together in teams or groups, a resident wisdom exists among them, and sharing testimonials is the way in which this wisdom is communicated.

Both through our work here in the United States and in our exploration of support and accountability in China, the power of the testimonial has become apparent. At the Cancer Recovery Society meetings in Shanghai, people's stories of recovery and their testimonials regarding their self-healing practice are their most powerful tools.

Medical treatment and the scientific proof for their self-healing practices are secondary. At one meeting following an hour of Qigong (Chi Kung) self-healing, I asked, "Do you feel there would be some value in doing some scientific research to prove the effectiveness of these methods?" Here is the answer: "While we are learning to practice the self-healing methods, we hear from dozens of people who nearly lost their lives to cancer. But they are alive and recovering. Over time, along with our daily practice we hear the testimonials of more and more of our recovery friends every day. We do not need science; our living friends are all the proof we need." The Cancer Recovery Society has convened two international scientific conferences, so they actually are exploring the scientific aspect of the issue as well.

Hearing the stories of others regarding their experiences with the self-healing methods or their breakthroughs in seeking emotional balance or their breakthroughs in faith will assist you. And you will assist others by telling your story. The usual setting for testimonial is in groups that meet together. A new setting for the powerful sharing of testimonial is emerging on the Internet, where many types of support and learning groups interact.

Who Heals Whom

The great playwright George Bernard Shaw wrote, "People are always blaming circumstances. . . . The people who get on in this world are those who get up and seek the circumstances they want."

Certainly expert facilitation is of great value in specific instances. Great athletes will always have coaches. However, participating in the event and winning the gold medal can only be accomplished by the individual athlete. Corporate employees will always have bosses. But those who do well and advance in their work do so by actualizing their own gifts and strengths. No one should go without needed surgery. However, avoiding surgery by remaining healthy is possible only when *you* take action for prevention.

Natural resources, including vitality and awareness, are present in all humans; they are not reserved only for especially fortunate individuals. Those who are wealthy, those who are employed, or those who graduate from college do not have more or fewer of these profound inner resources. These assets are inborn, a wealth that is shared by all. For some reason, this power that we share has remained a secret. Now the secret is out.

A Formula to Accelerate the Healer Within

First we discovered the healer within and the four essential methods for turning the healer on. The first simple formula of self-healing and health enhancement was noted in chapter 1 (page 96):

Awaken the medicine within, restore the natural self-healing capacity of the body, mind, and spirit.

Now we can add to this formula what we have just learned to create a more comprehensive and powerful self-healing formula:

Cultivate the influence of positive emotions, such as joy and gratitude. Cultivate the influence of positive attitudes, such as hope and accountability. Cultivate the influence of faith—faith in the "mystery," faith in science, and faith in what you have discovered yourself. Cultivate humor and fun. Neutralize anxiety, frustration, and fear. Seek the support of others, and serve others by supporting them. Listen for the stories and testimonials that confirm your inner potential to reach your preferred conditions and circumstances.

How can I do this when I feel weak, overwhelmed, or oppressed? When emotions, attitudes, or circumstances are holding you down, the first and easiest step is to take several Essential Breaths (page 86). Begin to massage your hands and then your ears while you keep the breath full and relaxed. Add one or several of the body movements. Use Spontaneous Movement (page 51) and Sigh of Relief (page 92) to shake free from fear and fuel your courage. Make sounds. These actions trigger the healer within. It is true that your case is unique and unusual. There are real reasons why you are in your situation. However, with the energy that you spend feeling like a victim and trying to find an expert to fix or cure the problem, you could heal yourself.

If you find that you are stuck and can't contact the healer within, find a group of others who are working with self-healing. The support, learning, and accountability available from a group are very powerful. Listening to the testimonials of others is healing in itself.

The self-healing and health enhancement practices alone are powerful. The practices multiplied by your belief, your joy, your calm, your faith, and your forgiveness create a tremendous holistic self-healing program that honors body, mind, and spirit. When you do your self-healing methods in a positive mental and emotional state, the biological effect is greatly magnified. When you use these tools vigilantly, you command the most profound medicine ever known in human history.

When Healing Includes Passage from This Life

Here is one of the most extraordinary lessons I have learned in over twenty years of medical practice. Usually it is taught by a person experiencing a severe or terminal disease.

It is not guaranteed that the person who lives the longest is the winner of the game of life.

One very excellent study on Qigong with cancer patients from Wuhan, China, reported positively on the "curative effect" of Qigong. Then, in the text of the abstract, there is this haunting line: "The unsurvivors passed away without suffering. Qigong practices play an important role in euthanasia for cancer patients."

It would be remiss to complete this chapter without telling the story of one of the people who taught this to me. Now she gives this teaching to you as well: surrendering to death is also a self-healing practice.

Charlene had used the health enhancement and self-healing methods in many forms throughout her life. She was a mom, a massage practitioner, and a community-minded person, not some-one who seemed likely to "die before her time." Being a health in-structor, health professional, and spiritual seeker did not spare Charlene from breast cancer, which eventually metastasized to the bone. Ultimately, she came to realize that her departure from this life was inevitable.

Over the years Charlene had developed her own personal ap-proach to the practice of self-healing. Now she purposefully turned her intention toward a kind of euthanasia in which self-healing became part of her life completion process. She had sup-port from hospice workers, a network of devoted friends, and expert medical assistance.

She added to the self-healing methods by deepening her spiri-tual practice. When she moved beyond the fear of losing her life, her faith expanded. When she realized that her resistance to losing her life was draining her vitality and making her condition worse, she began to explore surrender. This led to the essence of forgive-ness: forgiving oneself. She became calm, like a wisdom teacher. People commented that she was beginning to look radiant.

When it became impossible for her to continue the movement practices, she used the breath practice, deep relaxation, and med-itation. When she could no longer massage herself, she received massage from family and friends. She predicted the day of her passing several weeks before it occurred. She and her family had many fond memories of the summer solstice and the festivity of the annual solstice parade. She gently released her last exhalation on the morning of the solstice parade, as she had predicted she would.

Charlene taught many people a powerful lesson on how peaceful leaving this life can be. Because of her wisdom, her prac-tice of self-healing included faith, forgiveness, and surrender. She left a great message for her family and friends: death is not fright-ening or unkind. Genuine healing doesn't ask that we cheat death; it asks only that we live honestly.

CHAPTER 12

The Possible Community

*It is a primary characteristic of the superior
person that his or her practice of self-cultivation
is focused upon helping everyone in the society.*

Confucius,
Chinese philosopher, 500 B.C.E.

HEALTH IMPROVEMENT AND SELF-HEALING ARE EASIER
than we all imagined. Obviously, anybody can do these practices.
Now here's another surprise: these methods have hundreds of diverse applications right in your own community.

Allow me to take you on a tour of a possible community,
where well-being is a communitywide priority. We'll call it Radiance. This is how your community could look in the near future.
When health is intact, wellness activities take place at home and
throughout the community. When health has been lost, similar
programs are available at clinics, agencies, and the hospital. This
could be any community, large or small, American or European.
In some ancient cultures, a similar picture, in a less sophisticated,
smaller, and more natural setting, existed thousands of years ago.
As we go, imagine how you would modify the practices in part 2

of this book to work in these situations. Following this tour, look for another, very hopeful surprise. Every time you think, "This is impossible, all of these things could never happen"—just relax, be tranquil. You will find good news.

When Health Is Intact

As we look around the community of Radiance, you will be astounded by the many different environments in which the health enhancement methods have been implemented. The community has been purposefully participating in a nationwide trend known as the "Healthy Communities" movement for a number of years.

Home

You can peek in through the windows of the homes in this community or over the fence into the yards and find family members using the health enhancement methods in many ways. There is no age limit. Grandparents tend to practice more slowly, but they have more time. They use the methods to prevent arthritis, foster sleep, and sustain energy.

Teens transform dancing into health enhancement by remembering the value of relaxation and tranquillity as they rock to the beat of their favorite music. Teens have found that it is easier to study when they meditate daily. Self-esteem has increased while drug use and unwanted pregnancies have decreased, because stress mastery classes have helped kids use relaxation in order to think clearly before they act.

Small children use deep breathing to channel their excited energy and act like animals—deepening the breath and making animal sounds. Moms and dads use the practices to reduce work stress and sustain vitality. Many of the residents of Radiance, even some of the younger children, have learned to meditate or use deep relaxation daily. Almost everyone remembers to breathe deeply and relax as they fall into sleep and as they arise to greet the day. Everyone has discovered the benefit of these methods to avoid colds and flus.

School

At the community schools regular practice of the health enhancement methods is fostered for both students and teachers. Teachers are reminded consistently that their health insurance rates will be reduced if they use the doctor and hospital less often. Because the teachers and staff have been so successful at sustaining their high level of wellness, their insurance premiums have begun to go down. In the nationwide accounting of school health care expenses, this community's schools have gained top honors for several years. In practical terms, this has cut medical costs, and these cuts have been translated into increased retirement benefits for the teachers.

The health enhancement methods have been found particularly effective in several aspects of school life: academic performance, student behavior, and sports improvement. Students are, of course, encouraged to use the methods at home as well.

Students find that practicing the health enhancement methods increases wakefulness for study and mental coordination for learning. It has been discovered that students with learning deficiencies suffer less frustration when the methods are used to balance brain coordination and modify the body chemistry. In the special education classes, teachers use the methods playfully, vigorously, and frequently, as often as four or five times throughout the day. This has helped improve both the learning capacity and the attention spans of developmentally challenged children.

The school psychologists and counselors have been pleasantly surprised to find that students with behavior difficulties, either in or out of school, change as they learn to use the practices. Crime has declined among student offenders. Far fewer students are sent to the principal because of their behavior, and detention hall is less crowded. There is a "health team" meeting (a mentoring program) that students can elect to attend instead of detention. The problems associated with student frustration have decreased, and the benefits of elevated self-esteem have begun to emerge.

In sports the health enhancement methods have been used, as with Olympic athletes, to improve performance. Meditation and breath regulation improve endurance and focus. Self-massage prevents injury and speeds recovery times. The gentle movements are used to enhance internal vitality and improve small-muscle coordination. In addition, the music, art, and theater instructors all use the methods to support the creative process.

The student health office uses the methods with students who have medical complaints, frequently reducing the need for medication. The hospital and several local businesses have formed collaborative programs with the school to enhance the community's health status. The first use of the health enhancement methods at the schools was in connection with the regional "Healthy Community" project.

Business

Throughout Radiance—at the banks, at grocery stores, and in the larger corporations—the health enhancement methods are a prominent aspect of efforts to increase productivity and reduce medical expenses. Most of the businesses have in place either a wellness program or a continuous improvement process for work effectiveness. Several have both. The business community in Radiance has collaborated enthusiastically in the regional "Healthy Community" project.

The wellness programs use the health enhancement methods to complement smoking reduction, weight loss, and high blood pressure reduction activities. In each of these areas people are giving something up: cigarettes, snacking, salt. The health enhancement methods give them something to add, something to share. There are support and study groups associated with each of these aspects of wellness; through the groups, people learn to integrate lifestyle, attitude, and self-healing practices in order to produce the greatest health improvement possible.

The improvement efforts at several of the corporations have organized employees in teams in order to enhance their ability to create their product or render their service. People who use the methods tend to manage stress more effectively, have more energy and endurance, and miss fewer days of work each year. Team members often elect to begin or end their team meetings with a few of the health enhancement methods.

Many of the businesses in Radiance are using an innovative program called the "digital desk doctor." An individual's computer can be set so that an alarm rings to trigger a Remembering Breath (page 89) or a Momentary Method (page 122). It can be set to bring onto the screen, every forty-five to sixty minutes, a brief instructional graphic about one of the other health enhancement methods.

Also on the computer, the individual can access an information file called "quick cures" for colds, sore throat, headaches, constipation, allergies, and drowsiness; here, home remedies and herbal formulas are suggested to complement the self-healing methods. In addition, it just takes an instant to be linked to Internet sites where an immense amount of information on healing and personal vitality enhancement can be accessed and printed out.

The health insurance companies for the corporations in Radiance have begun to lower their premiums because the number of heart attacks and other serious and expensive medical episodes has decreased. Doctor visits for common ailments have decreased as well because employees have better skills for avoiding colds and flus as well as for accelerating recovery. An innovative system for tracking personal goals as well as medical visits (see PHASES, pages 246 and 257) helps employees understand how they are either sabotaging or improving both their health and their insurance costs.

Several of the larger companies actually provide their own insurance funding (called self-insurance). They have also started gainsharing programs. This is where participants get part of their annual health insurance money back if their health is excellent. People in these programs have become especially avid practitioners of the health enhancement methods. There is one particularly innovative program where an individual who naturally tends to have healthy behaviors is teamed as a mentor with an individual who aspires to improve his or her health. The training for the mentors (see pages 239 and 257) includes extra exposure to the health enhancement methods. The mentor helps teach the person with whom he or she is working how to integrate new behaviors that will improve that person's quality of life.

Senior Centers

Several of the places in the community where seniors gather have implemented health enhancement practice sessions. The elders of the community love these sessions for many reasons. The health enhancement methods help to reduce their need for doctors and medicines by improving their health status; they provide a focus for social interaction, which also increases the elders' health; and they support the time-honored role of seniors as the wise elders of the community.

There are several programs that use the health enhancement methods for specific health problems. There is the anti-arthritis group, the reduce blood pressure group, and the anti-aging and longevity group. Quite a few of the health improvement support groups use a lifestyle assessment (PHASES) to target strengths and weaknesses. There is spirited interaction among the seniors as they learn about improving their health and explore their choices in the area of attitudes, emotions, and lifestyles.

Seniors had grown tired of waiting until they were sick and then sitting around in doctors' offices waiting to get prescriptions for drugs that didn't always help their problem. Now their physicians are celebrating because they can concentrate on more difficult cases while having to deal with fewer problems caused by the side effects of medications.

The senior centers have begun to incorporate the health enhancement methods with numerous other activities: as warm-ups before the ballroom dancing sessions, for example, and in many of the fitness classes. They also offer a half-hour session every day before the senior lunch program and even before the afternoon lecture series. A number of enthusiastic seniors have begun to gather in the parks for practice sessions, insisting that they enjoy doing the practices in nature more than indoors. Several of these elders have started a program for teaching the methods to small children in day care and kindergarten.

The health enhancement methods have always been a focus for the wise elders of ancient cultures. Many of the seniors have taken up the study of Yoga from India. Others have taken up Chinese Taiji (Tai Chi) and Qigong (Chi Kung). It is not unusual to find the elders discussing references to freedom from worry and fear in the Bible and in other sacred traditions. Lively debate on the nature of healing, different meditation systems, and the effect of health enhancement throughout the community is common among the senior community.

The Hospital and Health Enhancement

The hospital has become very involved with the community's health. Many of the community's most successful health enhancement and wellness programs are supported by the hospital. Some of the community's first programs in the self-healing and health enhancement methods were cosponsored by the hospital and the community continuing education program.

The hospital staff's own wellness program has a strong link to their self-insured health insurance program, much like that of some of Radiance's corporations. The better the hospital staff does at maintaining their own health and reducing medical visits, the less their insurance premiums cost. The hospital has done a remarkable job of informing employees of the financial rewards of increased health. Most of the hospital staff—from the director, the doctors, and the nurses through the house and grounds staff—have had thorough training in the health enhancement methods.

Wellness is also linked to the staff's continuous improvement and productivity enhancement programs as well. As the hospital has had to accomplish more with less staff in lean times, the health enhancement methods have been excellent stress mastery tools. Some of the people at the hospital call the practices their "survival methods" because they have been so helpful during times of extreme stress.

When the hospital work teams have their meetings throughout the week, they often elect to use some of the health enhancement methods to open or close the meeting. When tempers are hot or when frustration and stress are barriers to progress, the methods are sometimes used to release tension. The Spontaneous Movement (page 51) with Sighs of Relief (page 92) is particularly effective to blow off steam and refocus the discussion. When the team has reached a goal worth celebrating, the methods, usually a brief meditation, are included in the affirmation of success.

The hospital has also collaborated with local businesses and corporations, the schools, and the churches to foster a wide variety of wellness programs. Any innovation that can help the members of the community understand the value of caring for and protecting their health gets the complete support of the administration and staff at the hospital. This sometimes includes financial support from the hospital's nonprofit foundation, as well as the frequent use of meeting space and staff support for activities that include the health enhancement methods. Several of the retired physicians and a number of the nurses are particularly involved in classes that teach health enhancement at the hospital, in the parks, through the adult education program, and at the community recreation centers.

The Parks

People tend to want to do the health enhancement practices in natural settings. Fortunately, the community of Radiance had the foresight to create and preserve several beautiful parks many years ago. These parks have become gathering places for all sorts of health enhancement activities. Originally, small groups began to meet in the parks on Saturdays and Sundays. Now practice groups meet throughout the week. Many of the people practice by themselves, usually facing the mountains, a body of water, or some trees. It is not unusual to see people doing the Gathering Breath (page 96), reaching out and gathering the healing energy from around them.

Most of the activities in the park are free. A number of the more experienced practitioners take turns leading the practices. Several members of the elder community lead early morning practice sessions and then linger to participate in discussion and sharing afterward on benches and at picnic tables near the ponds and streams. A few groups have begun to practice Taij; its 108 movements take real devotion to learn.

It is amazing to find so many different kinds of people of various ages involved in the health enhancement methods here in the park. This is particularly true on weekends, when people who generally practice alone at home before work come out and join the groups in nature.

Weekly Group Practice

There are many weekly group practice sessions throughout the community. However, there is one community-wide practice session that happens at the central park. People from all different segments of the community attend this session. During the comfortable warmer months the practice is held outside. It moves inside the park's meeting hall during the winter.

The teaching of this weekly practice is a collaborative effort taken on by a number of the teachers of the self-healing methods from throughout the community. They have agreed on a core practice that is repeated each week. In addition, for fifteen to twenty minutes prior to the concluding meditation, they each share something new or unique.

This weekly session is like a heartbeat in the community—it is always there, every week. It is designed to be completely flexible. Some people come every week. Others come on an occasional basis. People feel that this practice session helps them keep their personal practice going strong. Those who have been coming for five or six years comment that they learn something new or deepen their practice in some way at each weekly session. It is obvious to everyone that practicing in a group has a special effect.

Continuing Education and Community Recreation

Many of the programs sponsored by the community recreation department and the local adult education program have incorporated the health enhancement methods. The first self-healing programs in the community were cosponsored by the hospital and the regional continuing education program. Now the community recreation department provides space for the popular community practice session that happens every week.

Numerous evening adult education classes provide instruction in the health enhancement methods as well. Some focus the practices on specific areas like healthy pregnancy, cancer and stroke prevention, and eyesight improvement. Others just provide an hour or so of general practice. The dance, acting, and choir classes have all begun to use some of the practices to stimulate creativity and reduce injuries.

Fitness Centers and the YMCA

For many years the fitness centers and the YMCA had focused primarily on aerobics classes and weight training. Then they began to offer low-impact classes as well as variations on Yoga and Taiji. The fitness centers were among the first in the community to begin adding self-massage and brief meditations to some of the classes.

Because all sports performance is improved by mental focus, the centers have been offering classes in meditation and visualization for runners, swimmers, and even the basketball crowd. Self-massage has become typical as a part of the warm-up and cooldown for more vigorous exercise. Recently, a special class in various deep breathing methods has become quite popular.

Churches and Synagogues

The churches and synagogues in the community of Radiance have been most enthusiastic about the use of the self-healing methods. In earlier historical periods the church was often a source for healing and medical care. In the nineteenth and twentieth centuries the focus of healing shifted from the religious community to the scientific community. The churches fell into the background of healing.

Now there is a resurgence of the concept of the "healing ministry" in the religious community. All denominations have begun to develop "health and healing ministries." It has also become popular for the churches to sponsor "parish nursing" programs. A nurse is hired, generally part time, to interact with parishioners, to help the sick, and to create disease prevention and fitness programs.

All of the parish nurses in Radiance are active in teaching the self-healing and health enhancement methods. The concept of health assessment and group learning to improve lifestyle choices and mental attitudes is used along with the self-care methods and a busy mentoring program. The community has gained national media attention because the health-ministry programs in the churches have been so effective in enhancing the overall health status of the community.

The University

The University of Radiance has an impressive wellness center. It has combined conventional fitness and lifestyle assessment with health improvement teams, support groups, and student health enhancement councils. The focus on health and empowerment has fostered increased self-esteem and communication skills and is helping to improve general health, adaptability to stress, and academic performance.

The student health center uses a computer lifestyle assessment as part of an annual health fair every fall. Students who use the assessment and participate in a brief "health team" training program get reduced rates on clinic visits, wellness activities, the bookstore, and tickets to sports events and concerts. The discounts are particularly motivating, and a high percentage of the students participate. Many of the students meet friends at the health team training whom they keep throughout their college years. This program has a mentoring component that matches incoming students with older students who help to foster healthy behaviors from the beginning of the college experience.

The wellness center on the campus is right next to the fitness center and gym. Conventional athletics are integrated with activities that focus on meditation and self-applied massage. Various approaches to the health enhancement methods are popular with the students. It is common to see students doing shoulder massage for each other and even meditating together. Several classes in more advanced forms of health enhancement—Qigong, Taiji, and Yoga—have become quite common, too.

The staff of the wellness program and the campus health office have tracked statistics and find that the presence of wellness programs and the practice of health enhancement methods have had a positive effect on self-esteem and academic progress while helping to reduce the use of drugs and alcohol and the incidence of unwanted pregnancy on the campus. The physiology department has been doing some research on the health enhancement methods as well. They have found that the most likely reason for health improvement is due to the positive effect of the self-healing methods on neurochemistry, metabolism, and the immune system.

The health insurance for professors and staff of the university offers a significant gainsharing rebate for people who reduce their need for medical visits. The academic departments, administration, and facilities employees all operate as teams. They use the same health assessment as the student program. The health enhancement methods are widely practiced among the university staff, both privately and as part of group activities.

When Health Has Been Lost

The hospital has been particularly innovative in bringing the self-healing practices into an integrated relationship with medical care. This has also been true at the physicians' offices and clinics throughout the community as well as in agencies that deal with specific diseases.

When disease was the primary focus of medicine, physicians had to differentiate the diagnosis and treatment of patients very carefully. Medicines for one disorder are not suited—and frequently not safe—for another disorder. Now that the focus of medicine has shifted to include self-healing and health enhancement, it has been discovered that all diseases can benefit from self-care. While very carefully differentiated strategies must be used for different diseases in medicine, the same self-healing practices are beneficial in all cases.

The Clinics and Physician Practices

Because the citizens of Radiance have had so much exposure to health enhancement and self-healing throughout the community, it has been easy for the doctors to become involved in promoting wellness programming. In the past, physicians had become frustrated in their attempts to promote healthy behavior. People just expected doctors to fix them. Now that the self-healing methods are being used in schools, businesses, and even churches, their clients have become more familiar with the idea that self-care and self-healing are really useful.

Most of the physicians' offices and the clinics offer group support and study where lifestyle, attitude, and self-healing are combined. Specialty clinics for heart disease, cancer, arthritis, weight loss, birthing, fertility, depression, and so on offer group meetings where participants explore the effect of their emotions, attitudes, habits, and behaviors on health and disease. The same lifestyle assessment and health improvement system that is used in the businesses is used at the clinics as well. All of these group activities weave the self-healing practices into their meetings.

The doctors themselves do not have to become experts in wellness, health promotion, group support, or self-healing. These activities are implemented through nurses, health educators, occupational therapists, and so on. In most cases the doctors reflect briefly with their clients on wellness, support, and self-healing as they review the client's chart. In this way physicians become wellness doctors without having to become wellness experts. Their customers are happy because their doctor shows interest in their self-care activities. The doctors are relieved because they can become self-healing advocates while sustaining their focus on being medical experts.

It has been discovered that the patients, probably better called students, can actually do these health-based activities on their own. Many of the physicians' offices have instituted mentor programs. These are similar to the mentoring programs found in Radiance's businesses, schools, churches, and synagogues. The programs operate like a buddy system, where former patients help new patients learn and incorporate self-healing into their lives. These activities do not always happen at the physicians' offices or clinics themselves; they have also been implemented at the library, schools, churches, and community recreation facilities.

The earliest use of self-care in the community was in several of the natural healing clinics. The osteopathic physician, a chiropractor, and several doctors of traditional Chinese medicine had begun support or study groups and were encouraging the self-healing practices long before the hospital and other agencies started to do so. There is also a massage school in the community that was one of the earlier organizations to emphasize self-care and self-healing.

Agencies

The Heart Association, the Lung Association, the Cancer Society, the Multiple Sclerosis Society, the Diabetes Association, the Arthritis Association, and other agencies that work with specific diseases have enthusiastically supported a community-wide implementation of wellness activities. All are supportive of the regional "Healthy Community" project. Because each disease is a completely different entity, each of the agencies has had a long history of working in isolation to serve its clients. Now, however, because health enhancement and self-healing are the same for all people regardless of their diagnosis, the agencies have begun to collaborate in the areas of wellness, study groups, and self-healing practices.

An innovative new model of group support and study has emerged. Formerly multiple sclerosis support and diabetes support were separate, unrelated; now wellness-based support and learning activities have begun to accommodate individuals with various disorders in a single group. Because the participants have different disease challenges, they share less about doctors and medicines than in support groups that are specific to a certain diagnosis. Instead, they now focus more on personal healing strategies.

Another powerful feature of group support and study has emerged as well: peer-based group activity. Some of the group activities occur without an official or expert leader. Participants take turns being the facilitator for a weekly meeting. Each person has a chance to lead the self-healing practices during the group meeting as well. Mentoring is very common in this program.

The agencies found that they could collaborate to apply for grant money for these programs because, for the first time, they all had the same goal. Instead of being managed by any one of the agencies, there is a special office at the United Way where collaborative health enhancement activities are addressed. People with various diagnoses have access to the programs that are held at the library, hospital, school, community recreation centers, and continuing education facilities. The community self-healing practice session is a central gathering place for people from all of the agencies, in addition to those who are well. The weekly practice session is also managed by the collaborative office at the United Way.

In the social agencies that serve less fortunate populations, an innovative program called "Well Fare Plan for Well-Being" has started a new trend for families on welfare. Using the peer group method for personal improvement, individuals who are currently unemployed participate in a review of their lifestyle, attitudes, and self-care. The health enhancement methods are used at the beginning and the end of the peer group sessions.

Participants learn to facilitate the group, gain knowledge about health, vitality, and endurance for themselves and their families, and grasp basic skills for building self-esteem and creating a career plan. The businesses and agencies involved in the "Healthy Community" project have created a pathway for individuals who complete the "Well Fare Plan" to train for jobs that will become available in the near future. When openings become available, the participants transfer directly from the "Well Fare Plan for Well-Being" into a personal improvement group in their new company.

Self-Healing at the Hospital

The health enhancement and self-healing methods are prominent in numerous programs at the hospital for people who struggle with regaining lost health. Each of the disease management departments strongly urges people to use the self-applied health enhancement methods. The comprehensive cancer program, the cardiac rehabilitation program, the stroke recovery program, the diabetes program, and the occupational medicine department all teach and encourage the practice of the self-healing methods. Psychologists and social workers at the hospital typically urge their clients to practice self-healing and to work with a health mentor.

Several of the agencies throughout the community use the meeting rooms and the auditorium at the hospital for their peer groups and self-healing practice sessions. Recently, the hospital sponsored an immensely popular lecture and weekend workshop on self-healing and natural medicine. The mayor was there, and administrators from public schools and key people from most of the community's businesses and churches came as well. The event was a benefit to gather funds for the conversion of a wing of the hospital into the Integrated Natural Medicine and Health Promotion Department.

This project has been gaining momentum for several years. Primary care physicians and doctors of natural healing methods have been cooperating successfully to treat difficult cases and integrate services on general medicine and wellness without a central facility. With the new facility, this broad array of services will become available in one convenient location.

This program is an example of the community-wide commitment to a vision of a health care delivery system based on health enhancement rather than on disease treatment. Everyone has agreed—from the doctors to the administrators to the citizens themselves—that the new health center must have personal health enhancement as its foundation. A portion of the health care dollars that are saved when this program succeeds at reducing expensive surgical procedures (cardiac bypass typically costs $50,000 to $100,000), will be directed by a citizen panel into community improvement funds for schools, parks, and libraries.

The Politics of Health

The citizen advisory councils for both the Healthy Community project and the Natural Medicine and Health Promotion project urged the city council and the administrators to commit to a vision of community-wide cooperation to increase health and cut medical costs. Following this recommendation, the city council placed an initiative on the ballot. It was, as far as they can tell, the first of its kind in the country.

It reads: "We, the citizens of Radiance, resolve to participate in striving to make our community the healthiest community in the nation. In our schools, businesses, places of worship, and homes, we will take action to prioritize health improvement for the betterment of our community now and in the future."

The community wholeheartedly supported the initiative. It was one of those rare ballot issues in the voting history of the county that had no significant opposition.

Healthy Community Vision

Several years ago a number of businesses, schools, churches, and government organizations began a collaborative project to discover how to improve community health. First, they looked at how to improve medical services. They realized that medicine was addressing people only after they had lost their health. Then they looked at what services were not provided in the community. Several necessary services for children were missing, and the community worked together to fill those gaps.

Finally, they realized that the main issue in enhancing health was to help citizens access knowledge and tools in order to sustain their health, so that medical services would be less urgently needed. It was at that point that the peer group activities and the health enhancement methods became the prime focus of the "Healthy Community" project. The fund-granting organizations in the community helped to get self-healing and health enhancement methods practice sessions, health improvement teams, and learning groups going throughout the community. It is obvious from our tour of Radiance that this strategy has been a remarkable success.

Eventually, unofficial peer-based learning, support, and practice groups began to spring up spontaneously outside the clinics, agencies, and hospital. Casual groups have started among teachers at the schools, and small groups have begun throughout the senior community. There are singles groups, women's groups, professional groups. As people focus on learning about and improving their health, it is evident that it becomes easier to improve other aspects of their lives as well.

The "Healthy Community" project has sponsored the *Healthy Living* television show, which features tips on cooking, shopping, self-care, and wellness. There is a weekly sixty-minute self-healing TV program, "Healing Ourselves," that demonstrates the self-healing methods for people who cannot get out to the community practice session. People can access an Internet site where computerized libraries allow health information on self-care and suggested treatments for specific health conditions to be printed out. The site includes a directory of self-healing practice sessions, health-oriented learning groups, and self-care instructors.

Outcomes Measurement

One of the really important innovations in this community is that they have been tracking the results of their activities. Early in the "Healthy Community" process, the collaborating organizations decided to track several statistics to measure their success. They record and compare the number of hospitalization days, the number of corporate sick days, school attendance and academic skill levels, crime rates, citizen satisfaction with quality of life, and insurance company ratings for the community compared with the ratings of other communities.

Now that the program is several years old, these statistics are beginning to show that the community has made genuine progress in its health improvement efforts. A number of other communities have also been recording the same statistics. The race to become the healthiest community is on. At a recent international conference on community health, the mayor and the director of the hospital received a special award for the community of Radiance for its development of a comprehensive rating system for measuring community health status.

Is This Utopia?

This description is just a Utopian wish, you may be saying, the hope of an irrational optimist. Here is the surprise promised at the beginning of the chapter. In actuality, every one of the features described in this possible community is really in place somewhere. The community of Radiance is a composite of programs and activities that already exist.

Many of these actual hospitals, corporations, agencies, universities, and communities are among my clients who have implemented the SAHEM and PHASES programs in Ohio, Arizona, Washington state, Washington, D.C., Oregon, Minnesota, Florida, Michigan, California, Canada, Puerto Rico, and China. Others are sites I have visited. Many of these programs are already in place at businesses, agencies, and clinics in your own hometown.

The wellness programs at both the University of Arizona and the University of Minnesota are incredible, and the University of

Wisconsin is the home of the National Wellness Institute, which has sponsored over twenty annual wellness conferences. Motorola, Westinghouse, General Electric, and other corporations have award-winning wellness programs. Many have received the C. Everett Koop award from the Health Project that was originally founded by the White House and former surgeon general C. Everett Koop.

The "peer support" and "wellness" programs at the Multiple Sclerosis Society along with programs at the heart, lung, arthritis, diabetes, and other organizations have become very wellness-oriented in many communities. HIV organizations have been particularly open to self-care and alternative medicine. Many community-school systems have implemented all or part of the program described in Radiance. And right here in my hometown of Santa Barbara, the self-healing methods were originally implemented through a collaboration between the hospitals and the continuing education and city recreation departments. The Health Ministries and Parish nursing program of another Santa Barbara hospital just received a national award from the Catholic Health Association.

Radiance is not a fantasy; it is, however, fantastic. Nothing in the community described here is impossible or particularly complex. The cost to implement these activities is minimal, and no high-tech equipment is required. The most difficult obstacles to achieving this vision are our old habits and former thinking. People with vision and vitality can give reality in their own communities to activities like these with little more than willingness and enthusiasm. The idea that average folks in cities and towns throughout the world can't create this picture is an illusion. People can. In fact, people have.

The Keys to the Possible Community

How is it possible to create this kind of activity throughout a community? It is obvious that it is a fantastic concept. How can it actually work in our communities?

I have traveled to China five times to study their use of self-healing and health enhancement practices. I feel that there are some clues in China. The three areas of choice in health—attitude, lifestyle, and self-care—are a focus throughout Chinese culture. The medical system is not the foundation of healthy living. The wisdom of the ancients implemented through daily health enhancement practice is the foundation of the Chinese health care system. The medical professions and the Chinese government acknowledge and support this.

In China, then, the traditional keys to a healthy community include

1 Solo practice: Each person understands the benefits and values of daily health enhancement practice, which includes the health enhancement methods as well as keeping an even mental attitude and following basic wisdom in the area of lifestyle—diet, rest, hygiene, and so on.

2 Community practice: Communities provide facilities for public group practice in the parks, schools, and hospitals.

3 Community-wide support of traditional health wisdom: Government officials, business leaders, school administrators, physicians, hospital administrators—all are outspoken supporters of health enhancement. The community honors the teachers, mentors, and organizations who sustain the social vision of health throughout the community.

4 Mentoring: Teachers of the health enhancement methods are the most visible mentors. However, it is typical for average citizens to take on the responsibility of helping others to improve their understanding and practice of health enhancement and self-healing.

5 Traditional Chinese philosophy: With its ancient roots in the writings of Lao-tzu and Confucius, Chinese philosophy has supported these ideas for over 2,500 years. In China this system is built into the culture; it works automatically. In our own communities, it will have to grow and mature over time.

Sadly, this wisdom is fading in China among the younger people, who have been tempted by the material goals of Western societies. Happily, this wisdom is rapidly evolving in Western cultures, where the temptation of material goals has caused social, health, and economic problems.

The Chinese get Western medicine, the enterprise system of doing business, computer technology, hot water, and cars. The West gets acupuncture, herbal wisdom, meditation, self-healing, and philosophies that honor balance and harmony. Hopefully, this is a win for everyone. Community health enhancement promises to be an immense gift to Western culture. The gift of the awareness of the healer within may be one of the most profound breakthroughs in all of Western history.

There are clearly numerous American and European communities that have begun to enthusiastically implement health improvement activities. Fostering the health enhancement and self-healing methods is probably the most commonly utilized strategy for community health status enhancement in China.

Part 5

THE FUTURE

People did not weave the great web of life,
we are merely a strand in it. Whatever we do
to the web we do to ourselves.

Chief Seattle,
chief of Six Tribes of the White River

○

Each individual's willingness to take action to
sustain and improve his or her own energy
produces a powerful influence that has the
potential to affect healing throughout the
communtiy and even the world.

CHAPTER 13

What Could Be

*A human being is part of a whole, the
"universe." Our task must be to free ourselves
from the delusion of separateness, to embrace
all living creatures and the whole of nature.*

Albert Einstein,
physicist, philosopher

ONE OF THE MOST INSPIRING MOMENTS IN THE EVOLUTION
of the self-applied health enhancement methods (SAHEM) occurred at the annual conference of The HealthCare Forum, one
of America's largest hospital membership organizations. I had
been invited to do a presentation on the health enhancement
methods as an easy win for hospitals who wanted to take action to
improve community health status.

To highlight the diversity of people who could benefit from
the self-healing methods, I arranged for ten people of various
ages, races, health levels, and backgrounds from all over California to act as a demonstration team for the practices. Over 1,500
hospital executives, department managers, hospital trustees, and
medical directors were in the audience.

My message was that an easy way for hospitals and their communities to collaborate to enhance health would be to foster the

practice of health enhancement methods among people in businesses, schools, churches, and clinics. I was curious about the response that these leaders of the health care professions would have when I asked them to join in on some of the practices. When this idea came up in my lecture, a wave of embarrassed giggling and whispering went through the convention hall.

But when the time came, everyone was completely willing to participate. We started with the Flowing Motion done sitting, progressed to the Gathering Breath, and concluded with a brief meditation. Everyone participated enthusiastically and in perfect unison. The sight of so many people moving gently together was astounding. Only in China had I witnessed so many people practicing in such absolute unity. Three thousand hands rising and falling gently in perfect harmony looked like an expansive field of grain stirring in a summer breeze. During the meditation the quiet was immense.

Later several of the people I talked with declared that headaches and after-lunch indigestion had disappeared during the practices. But my biggest surprise actually came three months later at the annual conference of the National Wellness Institute. Following my presentation, Judy, the director of the wellness program at a large hospital in Kansas City, asked, "May I tell you about my experience at your demonstration at The HealthCare Forum?

"I'm sorry I missed the presentation. I walked in when you finished, just as the applause was beginning. I quickly became aware of a strange but very pleasant feeling, a kind of energy, I would say. I know you did some sort of exercise. It felt like a force field, very unique. In dozens of conferences in my career I have never perceived that feeling before."

There is a dynamic discussion emerging about healing and the mind, about energy healing, prayer, and new concepts in physics. The idea that a group of people practicing self-healing methods can create a beneficial influence or energy is new in Western cultures. In China, however, this idea is quite common. It is called the "healing energy field." I was delighted to hear Judy's impression. It suggested that even conservative executives and managers who might resist such a concept had still created a "field" so significant that it could actually be perceived.

Generating a "Field" of Healing Energy

The fact that a powerful healing resource is produced within the human system seems extraordinary enough. Yet there is another, even more phenomenal surprise: we produce a powerful healing resource among us as well. The name for this in China is *Qichang* (Chi Chang) *Gong*. It means "group-generated energy field with healing effect."

When groups practice self-healing methods together, the individuals in the group frequently experience an acceleration of benefits. This is common, something we've already explored. Qichang Gong goes way beyond what we know and understand regarding self-healing and group practice. The Chinese believe that each individual actually produces a personal "field" of healing energy. When groups of people practice together, these individual "fields" interact to produce a powerful "group healing field" (Qichang) that can beneficially affect persons who cannot do the practices themselves. I personally have witnessed this process, and it is a little like a kind of faith healing where an invisible spiritual presence is very strong.

The most famous and scientifically relevant example of Qichang Gong takes place at the Zhineng Qigong Hospital and Training Center, located in a former naval hospital in the mountains near Qinghuangdao in northeastern China, about five hours by train from Beijing. At this hospital there are usually over two thousand patients—but they are not called patients. They are called students because they are learning the lifelong skill of self-healing. The goal of Dr. Pang, the director of the hospital and the developer of the Zhineng Qigong concept, is to liberate people from their dependence on doctors and medicines and create health and endurance in the Chinese society. It is estimated that over eight million people practice Zhineng (which means "universal intelligence") Qigong (Chi Kung) throughout China.

When I discovered in 1988 that a doctor in China had a vision similar to my own, I began to plan to visit his center. At the second International Conference of Medical Qigong in Beijing in 1992 I received an invitation to visit Dr. Pang but was unable to arrange the details. Finally, through a string of coincidences, several connections in China, and the assistance of a Qigong friend, Luke Chan, the author of *101 Miracles of Natural Healing,* I was able to get special permission to visit Dr. Pang's Zhineng Qigong Hospital and Training Center in 1995.

I have had the opportunity to learn many forms of Qigong over the years and to visit many Qigong departments at hospitals, institutes, and temples throughout China, but I was especially struck by the enthusiasm of the practitioners at the Zhineng Center. The method itself is not complex, but the students earnestly practice Qigong almost all day. Sometimes whole families are involved in the program.

At the hospital there is no acupuncture, herbal medicine, or massage, all of which are typical in Chinese hospitals. There is no Western medicine, and there are no special healing diets. The only healing method is Qigong—self-healing. Those individuals who are severely ill or near death draw on the "group healing field." The ill or paralyzed person, either sitting in a chair or wheelchair or lying in a portable bed, is placed among the students who are practicing the self-healing methods in a group. Their practice intensifies or amplifies the "field" of healing energy. The immobilized students in beds, chairs, and wheelchairs bathe in and absorb the healing energy and imagine that they are practicing the methods.

Later, they begin to move their fingers, toes, hands, or feet while still sitting or lying down. Then more specific body movements are added as the person continues to absorb the healing energy created by the group. Eventually, strengthened by their own efforts and the "healing field," they recover enough of their vitality to join in the gentle movements of the group practice.

This fantastic process would be difficult for most of us in the Western world to accept. However, Dr. Pang is an innovative thinker as well as a hero and visionary to the Chinese people. He has been working for several years on documenting the results of Zhineng Qigong. There are several doctors at the Zhineng Hospital, but they do not give treatment. Their only job is to diagnose the students carefully on their arrival at the hospital, using modern Western methods like X-ray, CAT scan, ultrasound, and EKG in order to create a "clinical baseline." Following the students' stay and their practice of the Zhineng Qigong methods, the doctors complete a second evaluation to measure the results of their experience at the hospital.

Since 1988 the hospital has worked with many thousands of students with over 180 different diseases. The hospital has carefully measured the progress of a sample of eight thousand of the students (patients) and concluded in a 1991 report that 95 percent of the cases have had significant improvement (15 percent cured, 38 percent very effective, 42 percent effective; Pang, 1991). Many of these cases are students with cancer and paralysis. These astounding statistics, while inspiring, leave us with questions that require further observation: "How does Zhineng Qigong work?" and "How was the sample selected for the research?" As with the miracles and remissions that we explored earlier, for now it is particularly interesting that such a hospital exists and that there was improvement in 95 percent of eight thousand cases.

I can report from my own experience at the hospital that the zeal among the students is very high. Scientific evidence is of minimum interest to them. Their proof is the many people whom they have personally seen regain their health through this practice. They share testimonials throughout their stay at the hospital, and this strengthens the healing influence of belief. A number of people whom I was able to interview during my visit, particularly students who had become instructors, told of using Zhineng Qigong to recover from severe and "incurable" diseases.

The Zhineng Center is only one prominent example of this concept in China. Dozens of Qigong institutes have developed variations on the idea of a "group healing field." One might be tempted to think that the Chinese are just innocent, that they are not very sophisticated scientifically. But consider that the plow that started the agricultural revolution in Europe had already been invented in China 2,200 years earlier. This is an immense period of time. The Chinese realized the practical value of the decimal in mathematics 2,300 years before the concept found its way to Europe. Acupuncture, which many in the West still argue is a questionable clinical tool, evolved from the use of stone and bamboo needles in China around 3,000 years ago. It may be that this idea of a "healing field" is just another example of something the

Chinese will teach us in the West several thousand years after they discovered it themselves.

As we enter the fascinating realm of self-healing, it is exciting enough to discover that we can heal ourselves. But then to discover that in practicing together we can help to heal each other—this is an extraordinary revelation. Our independence frees us to heal ourselves. Then by simply shifting our intention, we can participate in generating a powerful influence that can benefit others.

Our interdependence, our sharing, and our cooperation magnify this strength. Together, it is possible for us to multiply our singular energies into an abundance. These effects are not wild imaginings; they are genuine aspects of the world we live in. Real people, multitudes of them, engage in these activities in China every day. How can we understand these possibilities? How shall we embrace this practice? How might we benefit from this radical breakthrough?

There Is an Energy

I have had the opportunity to share the health enhancement and self-healing methods with people in immensely varied situations—with health seekers at the clinic, with lecture and conference audiences, even with troubled individuals whom I have met on airplanes and commuter trains. In every case, when people break through to an experience of self-healing, it produces a powerful enthusiasm.

There is a dynamic energy in this enthusiasm that is tangible. And it differs from just interest or gratitude. Enthusiasm is actually defined as "inspiration from a divine or celestial source." Sometime around 1985, after fifteen years of my own practice, I found myself awakening to the possibility that the energy I was experiencing was an actual force that could be purposefully directed.

When this same energy is multiplied in groups, it becomes enchanting. It is discernible yet subtle, like a magnetic field. When Judy, the director of the Hospital Wellness Center in Kansas City, walked into the hall at the Anaheim Convention Center where over 1,500 hospital executives had just been practicing together, she was astonished to find this energy perceptible, palpable.

Through my study of Chinese medicine I learned that life and health are driven and sustained by a mysterious energy, the Qi (Chi). I had been assuming that this energy was within the person and that it could be affected by acupuncture and enhanced by self-healing practice. But then it became clear that the energy is not just within us. When I began to experience this energy with groups, it became not only a focus for investigation but a source of enchantment and a promise of something profound. I am sure that this energy has potential that we have only just begun to discover.

At the 1992 World Conference on Medical Qigong, I was privileged to visit the China National Radio and Television Research Laboratory in Beijing, where high-level exploration of Qi was in progress. With twenty other doctors and scientists I witnessed a tightly controlled experiment that demonstrated clearly that the body's "field" is not contained inside the skin.

Through sophisticated equipment, we observed that an individual in a chamber, completely sealed off from all outside frequencies, could emit energy over a distance. Before this I had practiced acupuncture for over fifteen years with exciting clinical results but had accepted Qi as only a possibility rather than a reality. When the equipment began to show an emission of energy from the research subject's body, my professional curiosity transformed into pure amazement. Following this impressive laboratory encounter, my experience with Qi (life force, vital energy, subtle energy, or natural healing resource) has rapidly accelerated.

The Qi is multiplied when people practice personal enhancement together in a group. Here is the moment of wonder; this is the sweetest, most spectacular possibility: as we move toward an understanding of the nature of "healing fields," we may find ourselves able to cooperate to produce healing potential that will help us to benefit one another.

Distance Is Not a Barrier

My most astounding experience with the fact that our healing influence may not be limited within us occurred in the winter of 1992. I received a call from a physician, a dermatologist in New

York, who said he had read some of my writing in the *American Journal of Acupuncture* (Jahnke, 1989) on the Chinese self-healing methods. He reported that his mother's health was deteriorating and that all of the possibilities for medical treatment had been exhausted. For several weeks she had been eating less and less and seemed to be losing her ability to recognize her son.

He asked sincerely if I felt there was really a chance that a healing energy could be extended across a distance to help others. I responded that I had witnessed some things in China and had some clinical experiences that suggested that such distant healing was possible. I noted several scientists and scientific associations that were actually studying this kind of phenomenon.

I was not expecting the doctor's next statement: "Will you send healing energy to my mother?" While my intellect was rushing to apologize and decline, my voice said that I would be willing, of course. After all, I do these practices every day, and there was really no reason to refuse. It was obvious that he was preparing himself for the passing of his mother; and I felt open to exploring his request. For the next several days I purposefully held the name of the doctor's mother in my mind off and on during my practice of the health-enhancing methods.

That Wednesday at the group practice session I mentioned briefly that we should allow our practice to have a distant benefit. I intentionally directed our influence to the doctor's mother. I was surprised to have a call from New York on Thursday morning. "Please, continue with whatever you have been doing," the physician said. His mother had improved over the last several days. On Wednesday afternoon and Thursday morning, he reported, she had actually talked to him lucidly, and her appetite was improving.

The Light of Science

Dr. Larry Dossey is my favorite among the contemporary explorers on this concept of a "healing field," which he calls a "nonlocal healing effect." His books, *Space, Time, and Medicine, Recovering the Soul,* and *Healing Words,* I feel, are among the most significant works of our time. He has gently turned the light of science on the mysteries of our spiritual traditions. In *Recovering the Soul* he describes a study with heart attack patients that supports my experience with the doctor from New York.

Randolf Byrd, a cardiologist, designed a study to explore the healing potential of focused intention or prayer (Byrd, 1988). The study involved 393 patients who were admitted to the coronary care unit of San Francisco General Hospital and were divided into two groups: 192 were placed in the "home prayer" group, and 201 in the "not remembered in prayer" group. The study was carefully designed according to the most rigid guidelines for research; therefore the findings are respected by scientists.

Each patient in the "home prayer" group had five to seven people praying for him or her. The "prayed-for" subjects had five times less need for antibiotics, were three times less likely to develop pulmonary edema, and were twelve times less likely to need artificial assistance with breathing (endotracheal intubation). These findings are not just mildly noteworthy; they are quite significant.

Dr. Dossey pursued his research further and found an organization called Spindrift that had asked two important questions (Owen, 1988): (1) Does nonlocal intention (prayer) actually work? (2) What kind of nonlocal intention (prayer) is most effective? These questions mirror two that I have had about the "healing field": Is there a "healing effect" outside ourselves? How is it best activated?

In numerous experiments on various biological systems, repeated many times, the Spindrift researchers found that nonlocal intention had a definite effect in enhancing biological activity. They found that when participants focused on a particular outcome, their success was actually less dramatic than when "nondirected" focus was used. In prayer of the latter type, the focus equates to the request that "thy will be done." In less religious terms this kind of nonlocal intention focuses on "the optimum," "the best possible outcome," or "the greater good."

These two examples and Dr. Dossey's work in general lend powerful support to the idea that we can have a positive nonlocal effect. Through our own solo practice, when intention is focused, our influence can affect others. In the Byrd study and in the Spindrift experiments, it did not matter whether those offering the prayers or focused mindfulness were together or apart. It did not matter what their religion was. Distance did not vary the results either. The implication is that the intention to have a positive influence is extremely powerful.

In Oakland, California, in 1994, twelve-year-old Alison Kuhn applied these principles to violence in the schools. She constructed an experiment on focused intention and prayer for the science fair at her school. During the month of February she asked students to pray for a reduction in the possession of weapons in the Oakland public school system. As a control group she used the schools in Berkeley, California. No one prayed for those schools. Oakland experienced a 66 percent reduction in weapons possession while Berkeley experienced an increase. Alison won the first prize at the science fair for her study.

Thank You, Dr. Einstein

A series of radical scientific breakthroughs that began with Albert Einstein help to lend credibility to the possibility of the "healing field." His general theory of relativity demonstrated that matter and energy—stuff and nonstuff—are interchangeable. This was in 1915, a long time ago. Unfortunately, this powerful information was used to build the atomic bomb, but it also has many benevolent applications, which include healing.

Among the many findings that have sprung from Dr. Einstein's original discovery is the concept in quantum physics that events can occur as either particles or waves. We have a refined sense of the particle world. Particular events can be seen, measured, and weighed. We have a less refined sense of events that manifest as waves. Electricity and magnetic force, as examples, are difficult to perceive, measure, or weigh. As another example, scientists discovered only fairly recently the energy (waves) that causes the heart to beat, but the heart itself (particles) was discovered thousands of years ago.

This is why medicine based on chemical drugs and surgical procedures, both of which address parts (particles), has a long history in the Western world, while energy medicine (waves), including acupuncture and homeopathy, has only recently gained favor. Our particle self has an "edge" or boundary; that is, it is local, substantial, and differentiated from others. Physicists who explore "relativity" and "quantum" physics have found that the wavelike or energetic aspects of ourselves are not separated in the same way; they are unfixed or undetermined. Our wavelike nature does not have an edge or boundary, is not limited to being local, is not substantial, and is not clearly differentiated from others.

In her fascinating book on this subject, *Quantum Society,* Danah Zohar explains this energetic, not substantial aspect of ourselves, which is not contained within the envelope of the skin, using the words "relational holism." The quantum side of our nature is part of a continuous, invisible "field" in which everything is interconnected and relational. "Beyond the always shifting boundary of the 'I,' relational holism draws the unfixed aspects of the self into ever wider circles of creative relationship—the intimate partner, the family, the group, the nation, 'humanity' itself" (Zohar, 1994).

This points to the fact that the quantum aspect of our self and ourselves has the potential to interact in a wavelike, undifferentiated interchange that occurs beyond the capacity of our particle nature (eyes and ears, for example) to perceive. David Bohm, the great contemporary physicist and philosopher, explained that it is when entities are in their wavelike state, an as-yet-undetermined state, that they can have a nonlocalized effect. Thus, when you are in the self-healing state where vital energies are dynamic and your mind is simply directed toward oneness, you can interact with "possibilities." You can connect with the wavelike, as-yet-undetermined aspects of yourself and others.

This is the healer within us activating a profound medicine among us. In our practice, we can elect with little additional effort to focus our wavelike nature through mind intention. Is disease an expression of our particle self or our wavelike self? The Chinese insist that disease is caused by a disharmony in the body's energy system, the wavelike self. Even Western science is clear that the heartbeat is an electrical discharge, that nerve impulses are ions discharging, and that the rate of movement of molecules through cell membranes is modified by energy charges. Can we help to heal, potentiate, or empower each other? Millions of Chinese believe that we can, and quantum science suggests that this notion from Chinese medicine is relevant and real.

Are crime and violence fixed and determined within our communities, or are they wavelike, as yet undetermined? Herbert Benson has proposed the idea that the "relaxation response" and meditation can have effects beyond physical healing in the area of behavior. In studies with students they have found that self-esteem increases in those who learn to meditate, with improved academic results and a significant decrease of inappropriate classroom behaviors.

What if gang members practiced the self-healing methods? If criminals had learned as children to do self-healing practices, would they have taken a different path? Would holistic living and stress mastery cause a decline in crime and violence? Can health enhancement build safer communities? The Edgar Cayce Foundation in Virginia Beach has sponsored a program for twenty-five years through the Association for Research and Enlightenment (A.R.E.) for inmates of prisons throughout the United States. The A.R.E. receives fifty letters a week requesting information about holistic living, nutrition, massage, meditation, and prayer. Many of the prisons have support and study meetings for group practice of meditation, breathing methods, and discussion of personal transformation.

Of their thousands of testimonials these three were especially expressive: "The A.R.E. program helped me find a new way of doing things" (Rick, thirteen years after release, Ohio). "Everyone in our study group made parole and never returned to prison" (Buster, thirteen years in prison). "I credit the Edgar Cayce principles for self-improvement as the turning point in my life" (John, eighteen years in prison, Pennsylvania). One prison psychologist reported, "This program is more effective than the official rehabilitation programs in meeting inmates' unique challenges."

The Wholistic Stress Control Institute in Atlanta works more proactively with this concept. Jennie Trotter, executive director, founded the institute in 1985 with violence, crime, and drug abuse prevention programs like "A Brother Is a Terrible Thing to Waste" and "Saturday Institute for Manhood and Brotherhood Actualization" (SIMBA). These programs use stress management, relaxation practices, massage, Taiji (Tai Chi) and wellness methods to foster transformation in self-esteem and personal belief systems.

The institute has won numerous awards from the Georgia governor's office and other statewide agencies. The institute has received recognition nationwide and taken the trainings to schools and communities in most states. "To me, recognition from the agencies is secondary," Jennie states, "to the feedback I receive from kids, relieved parents, teachers, school officials, and representatives of law enforcement." One of the parents said, "I believe this program saved my children's lives." Many of the school principals have been very impressed and believe the program should be taught in schools all over the United States.

Some particularly amazing research from the social science literature confirms the theory that the more people quiet their minds daily in a community, the less crime and disease will exist in that community. On the surface it seems logical, because anyone who uses deep relaxation practices daily will be more well, less affected by stress, and less likely to commit a crime. However, this theory suggests an even deeper benefit: those who are meditating create an effect or "field" that can influence even those who do not meditate.

During the war in Lebanon between 1983 and 1985 a study was done documenting an index of factors, including the number of war deaths and war intensity (Orme-Johnson, Alexander, 1988). It was predicted that if a large enough group of people were commited to shifting the "coherence within the collective unconscious" through meditation, the index factors would decrease, showing less violence. During seven test periods throughout the war the "coherence" group exceeded the necessary threshold for a worldwide effect. During these seven periods there was a composite average reduction of war deaths of 71 percent and a reduction of war fatalities of 68 percent.

A later study using the same methodology, meditation, found a similar outcome in the three major causes of violent death in America (motor vehicle fatalities, suicide, and homicide) during a similar period, 1982–1985 (Dillbeck, 1990). During the experimental period the size of the meditation group exceeded the necessary threshold for a national effect in 128 weeks, which correlated with an average decline of 106 deaths per week.

These findings and many others point to the fact that the practice of quieting the mind has an external effect that influences even people who are not in the meditation group. Somehow, benevolence, virtue, and healing are conducted within the "field." Fascinating debate has emerged from this kind of research. Is this effect due to an unknown characteristic of a known phenomenon like the electromagnetic field? Or is it due to a more pervasive and as yet unknown phenomenon like a "quantum field," the "unified field," or an all-encompassing "universal consciousness"?

The scientists at the Maharishi University of Management who did the research I've discussed on transcendental consciousness and Transcendental Meditation suggest the latter, in keeping with the ancient philosophical system from the Vedas of India. The ancient thinking of the Chinese Taoists would suggest that a pervasive transcendental effect is due to "original cause," often called the Prenatal Original Source or the Mystery. Both of these perspectives have presumed for thousands of years that there is far more to the world than what we know. And the physics community has now demonstrated that although in our particle lives we appear to be separate and individual bodies, in the wavelike sense we are all part of one universal body.

It is our good fortune in the exploration of self-healing, personal strength, and peace (reduction of crime and violence) that we don't have to wait until this debate is settled. It doesn't matter so much how the field works—the important thing is that it works. And excellent research in numerous fields demonstrates that the "healing field" is real. As more people become aware of what the honorable Einstein's work has revealed and practice using the field's effects, it will become easier to answer the questions that are so compelling to our scientists.

Those who practice self-healing methods, in addition to healing and empowering themselves, can have a positive effect on others. This influence flows to the sick as healing energy. The same influence may flow as benevolence and virtue to neutralize negative forces, like crime and violence. The effect that one can have on others requires little additional effort. Simply doing one's own practice in a state of benevolent intent is all that is required.

Possibility Formula for Producing a Medicine Among Us

This is a formula for something quite profound, a kind of blueprint for magic:

Personal practice generates creative energy, a field. The field effect is multiplied among all who practice. The field is an influential force. This influence heals. It is benevolent.

This concept is charged with potential. Excitement about these possibilities produces enthusiasm, which is an aspect of our wavelike nature. Enthusiasm connects us with the "divine," the "unfixed," and the "as yet undetermined." This multiplies the potential even more. Our intentional practice may link us to a wavelike field of possibility that could bring healing and virtue into the world. The potential of this concept is phenomenal.

When this energy is present, you can feel it. There is actually an awareness, even a sensation. Families, companies, or communities that generate this energy are magnetic. Perhaps you have said at one point or another, "I really like the feel of this town," "I was energized at that gathering," or "There is something special about the Jones family." We can use this powerful resource, this healing energy among us, to heal our communities.

Scientists and mystics agree: all of the universe is a single, unified field of interacting forces. In the quotation at the beginning of this chapter, Albert Einstein acknowledges that we are connected to the universe and that we must free ourselves from the delusion of separateness. Chief Seattle's haunting speech reflects the Native American understanding of this same uninterrupted unity of all beings and events in nature.

Earlier we discussed how it is a tragic oversight that we should produce a powerful healing resource naturally within us and then somehow forget to use it. Now we can take this a giant step further. It is astounding that we have the capacity to create a healing resource among us that we have not been using.

Is it possible that there is a nearly magical energy "field" that we influence while having the fun of doing our health enhancement practices? The answer appears to be yes. Why aren't we using this? Even when people do their practices individually, they multiply the potential for the whole. In addition to its application to healing, this energy can be used to redesign our lives, mend and rejuvenate our communities, and even transform our world.

Modifying Your Practice to Potentiate the Healing Field

Earlier we recognized that among the keys to the practice of self-healing and health enhancement, relaxation is primary. This is also the key to optimizing the "healing field." To participate in influencing this field, all you need do is either enter a state of meditation, as in the mindfulness and insight meditation (page 110), or add relaxation to your practice of self-massage, breath practice, or gentle movement. Then simply focus your attention in one of these two ways:

1 Specific directed focus
2 General undirected focus

The first focuses on directing the "field" specifically, as you do in praying for peace for a particular person, family, community, or country; the healing of someone in a certain situation; or for the safety of certain individuals or groups. The second affirms your alignment with universal wisdom and involves surrendering to or embracing divine order—simply celebrating what naturally occurs. Focus your intention on affirming the perfection of life, the order that prevails in the universe, or the presence of God's love.

Whichever path you choose, the effect is similar, although as we have seen, there is some evidence that undirected focus is the more powerful. By simply doing your practice and focusing your intention, you help to produce an influence that supports and benefits yourself and others. This profound possibility requires little extra effort in your practice, just the capacity to remember to focus your mind's intention.

An Abundance of Possibilities

Just so it is clear how multifaceted the act of simply doing your self-healing practice can be, allow me to review the effects that your practice of these health-enhancing methods can have:

1 *In solo practice:* The benefits and value for ourselves are always present. This is the key theme of this book. Solo practice is the path to independence and self-reliance. It is the foundation of all of the following effects.

2 *In solo practice:* Even though we might be alone, we are part of the larger group of those practicing self-healing throughout the community and even the world. This actually has two effects. First, when more people practice self-healing and health enhancement, each adds to the worldwide volume of health and peace of mind. This is like simple addition in math and is a marvelous strategy for community improvement. Second, each practitioner becomes a part of a larger "field" of influence that fosters health and peace of mind even in people who are not practicing. This is a more transcendental concept—rather like multiplication.

3 *In group practice:* The effect of our own experience is deepened or expanded. It is common for people to be aware of this effect and comment, "When I practice with a group, I am aware of an increased sense of well-being." This is a simple form of interdependence.

4 *In group practice:* The group produces a "healing field" that can benefit others who draw on this powerful resource to increase their vitality. The "field" can even influence those who are not involved in the practice, helping them to experience improved health or modified behavior. This is a marvelous form of interdependence that literally redefines our understanding of how the world works and may help to neutralize violence and crime.

There is something here for everybody. All of these point to a bright future. Rest in knowing that simply practicing will help you to heal or to enhance your health. For those who embrace and celebrate the "healing field" concept, rejoice in knowing that simply by doing your own practice, whether you are alone or with a group, you are emanating healing energy that can have a benevolent effect on your community and the world.

Health Enhancement, Self-Healing, and the Future

By creating a rebirth of self-reliance and mobilizing people to heal themselves, we make possible a brighter, better future. There are two approaches to thinking about the future that are recognized by experts in this area, generally called "futurists." In one, the future is forecast by noting current trends. In the second, the future is not forecast but designed by insightful and energetic people, drawing on vision and wisdom.

In the first we are at the effect of current trends, waiting for what will happen. In the second we are at the effect of our inspiration and imagination, literally creating what we hope for, crafting what could be. Gandhi, probably the greatest teacher of how to create a preferred future, left us this declaration on how to do it: "Become the change you want to see." With the richness of the human imagination and spirit, I have no doubt that a meaningful, exciting, and safe future is accessible.

Use and share these simple self-healing methods to participate in the seeding of a new era in health care and healing. Do this first in your own life, starting with the tools in this book. We can transform the future of health care and medicine by demanding that the system change. But this change cannot actually occur until we are willing to change ourselves from patients into students of health and vitality. You are the most important person in your health care and personal empowerment process, because only you can act daily and throughout the day to mobilize the potent resources within you.

All of the forms of self-applied health enhancement, whether ancient or new, are powerful tools for maintaining our health, nourishing self-reliance, cutting medical costs, and redefining the future. Whatever the method, the point is always the same: mobilize the healer within. In addition to movement of the body, massage, breath practice, and relaxation, carefully attend to right diet, sufficient rest, liberal intake of fluids, meaning and purpose for your life, engaging work, telling the truth, social interaction, humor, and having fun. These tools are time tested, they are always with you, they require no prescription, and they are absolutely free.

Healing the World

If each person were to embrace the simple ideals and tools that we have explored here, our world would be a dramatically different place.

When each person does the small job of taking care of himself or herself, the big job of taking care of everyone is automatically complete.

A new kind of health care and a new medicine are emerging that are founded in activating the healer within. Each of us is a key figure in the transformation of human possibilities. Healing oneself and helping others to understand the power of health enhancement: these are among the most honorable and powerful actions that anyone can take in these times.

As you have found through reading this book, the greatest resource for increasing health is produced within. If you will go ahead now and demonstrate this to yourself through personal action, you will have healed the piece of the world that you occupy. You are breaking free from the long-held misunderstanding that average people are not resourceful enough to do these things.

Then, if you accept the challenge to share these simple truths and actions with others, you become a kind of hero. Remind loved ones to take a deep breath, not by telling them to but by radiating your transformed self. Help co-workers to remember the value of simple self-massage by remembering to do massage for yourself. Teach the Momentary Methods to those around you by being someone whom people ask, "How do you stay so calm in the midst of complexity?"

It can be even easier than this, if you wish. You can simply act on these truths quietly, personally. Even if you keep your self-healing practice hidden like a "light under a basket," you are still refusing to be a part of the problem, and you become spontaneously transformed into part of the solution. As we have seen, just by shifting your attention slightly during your practice, you can also become a participant in the generation of a profound "field" of healing. Heal yourself and you heal the world.

Without even knowing each other, we cooperate toward a shared, positive consequence. Without even having to meet or plan, we can cocreate a powerful outcome. Through our quest for health, in our own personal practice, we bring into being a more healthy world. Through the peace that we seek sincerely within ourselves, we multiply the presence of peace in the world around us.

> Can you master your wandering mind
> and embrace original unity?
> Can you calm your breath, cultivate essential energy, and
> sustain the suppleness of a newborn with no cares?
> Can you clarify and refine your inner vision
> until you perceive nothing but pure, radiant light?
> Can you love without expectation or contrivance
> and guide others without imposing your own desires?
>
> Lao Tze
> Ancient Healing Formula, 500 B.C.E.

Appendix

Accepting the Opportunity to Share the Self-Healing and Health Enhancement Methods with Others

Some of you will become so enthusiastic about these possibilities for personal and community healing that your activity will overflow into service. Albert Schweitzer said, "To work for the common good is the greatest creed." Giving yourself to the service of others by sharing the self-healing and health enhancement methods is not complex. At the simplest level you can just share what you have experienced with other individuals who seem interested.

In every ancient culture these practices were taught by mothers and grandmothers to the children. Mentors teach students. Neighbors exchange family secrets. Even in modern America there are nonprofessional, community-based health experts. A great study by Eva Salber in Durham, North Carolina, found a system of "natural helpers" to whom people reached out before turning to their doctors (Salber, 1976). It is natural for guidance and teaching to be available in a community. Serving and sharing with others is an innate quality of human nature.

Decline the urge to judge or compare the people who accept the opportunity to share; just relax and do the practice. This is not a contest. The winner is not an expert. Celebrate the people who share their enthusiasm; they are heroes. This is a community-based revolution; it rests on the same ideals on which the American democracy is founded. The members of General Washington's army were humble idealists. But their most powerful tool was commitment to a vision.

The flag was sewn from simple cloth. A handful of devoted people swore allegiance to work together, and then, through their cooperation, they accomplished something profound that is still viewed with awe by people all over the world. In a similar spirit we can reinvent health care with a basis in wellness, health enhancement, and self-healing.

Community-Wide Practice Sessions

A weekly, community-wide practice session can provide a kind of heartbeat for everyone's independent practice. And it can be a heartbeat for community improvement as well. Find a centrally located facility with parking, bus access, and wheelchair accessibility. Make a simple proposal to use the space for a weekly gathering of citizens to practice health enhancement. The goal is to have people from throughout the community practice together for about an hour one day a week. Ensure that the space is available before and after the session so that the healing benefits of social interaction are woven into the design.

No one organization needs to sponsor this unless those who are responsible for the space require it. It is better to request that the space be free as a service to the community or at least quite inexpensive so that the practice session costs little to support. The Wednesday Self-Healing Practice Session in Santa Barbara charges participants five dollars a week. Just as it is important to keep your practice simple and fun, so it is recommended that your community practice session be easy and fun.

Every individual is unique in his or her practice; similarly, each individual community will find a unique way to create its weekly practice session. Solo and group practitioners from throughout your community will find out about this session. The self-healing group from the cancer center, the health enhancement group from the senior center, groups from other agencies, and individuals who are practicing because their doctors have encouraged them—all will be drawn to this weekly session.

The newspaper will notice what you are doing and run a story. Agencies will run notices in their newsletters. Then more people will come. The numbers will ebb and flow. People will get inspired and come often. Then their practice will become more personal and home based, and they will be out of the mix for a while. Later, they will return to the weekly sessions. Then they will go on a vacation or move away for a while. Months or even years later they will return and look for the practice session, knowing that it must still be meeting. If it is set up carefully, no one will own it and no one will have to come every time. It will always be there like a heartbeat in your community, a vital life center. It can be a basis for the renewal of self-reliance, health enhancement, and healing. All of this benefit, all of this possibility— yet there is little cost to anyone.

See "Resources" (page 257) for information on training and networking with other practitioners.

Teachers and Mentors

Many readers will want to share these health enhancement methods with others. The desire to do so is all that is required. The dictionary definition of "to teach" does not set restrictions on who can impart knowledge. Neither does the definition of "mentor" restrict who shall impart wisdom and counsel. There are natural instructors among you, and obviously, the health enhancement methods are not complex. My experience has been that in any community there are dozens of people who are eager to lead the group now and then.

Here in Santa Barbara a number of individuals have started up other practice sessions in addition to our regular Wednesday session. It is natural for people to want to share their personal practices with others. In China many of the teachers volunteer to repay whoever taught them by instructing the public. Such individuals are honored as cultural heroes. This is a fun and healthy way to do community service.

At the Zhineng Qigong Center and in the Cancer Recovery Society, which promotes Guo Lin's Qigong (Chi Kung), the method for targeting and training instructors is simple. Healed or recovered individuals feel strongly that it is their responsibility to repay the "system" for the gift of recovered health. Typically this repayment takes the form of teaching others. In numerous trips to China I have met over a hundred Qigong self-healing instructors who were motivated to teach by their own personal recovery from serious disease.

The teachers and mentors of self-healing practices are average people. They do not have to be doctors or educators. They are not health industry professionals. They are all simply individuals very much like you, who became interested in self-healing. They experienced the benefits of self-healing independence and then elected to give back, to pass the gift on to others through the path of interdependence.

Perhaps you recognize the opportunity for community improvement. If you feel called or if you feel compelled, you are the perfect teacher. Your enthusiasm and your story are your credentials. Your own experience with the methods will enrich your knowledge, and through your personal evolution in the practice your teaching will improve.

Dena, a psychotherapist in Maryland, has an interesting story. She is one of the most enthusiastic teachers and mentors I have met. She uses the self-healing and health enhancement methods with therapy groups, in workshops, and in her work with several social service agencies. In her work with an addiction recovery agency, she facilitates a practice session that is available to people in both the detox and the recovery phases of the program.

"The beauty of these methods is that everyone can benefit and everyone can become a teacher for someone else," Dena says. "One of the fellows in the program, a homeless man, while benefiting from the methods in his recovery from alcohol, also healed his knees following an accident. He was very good at leading the class in some of the self-massage practices for the knees. Another, a big man from the African-American community, told how he helped his mother with her arthritis by sharing the methods with his family."

One of my favorite teacher-mentors is Amelia in New York City. She took to the concept of self-healing quickly and completely. She works on Wall Street for an investment firm. In addition to her own practice, she has volunteered to teach self-healing in the HIV/AIDS community. She also meets occasionally with curious friends and acquaintances who wish to learn health enhancement methods in what she calls a "Qigong rendezvous."

Collaborative Departments and Agencies

One of the most powerful features of the "new" health care system is the focus on health improvement. Instead of requiring different programs for different diseases, as in medical intervention, health promotion is the same for all diseases. This means that programs or departments that formerly worked in isolation because of diagnostic differences can now collaborate.

Health care institutions can look at the possibility of bringing clients with heart problems, cancer, diabetes, multiple sclerosis, arthritis, lung disease, HIV, chronic fatigue, and so on together in programs based on health improvement and self-care. This requires a change in how the individual departments interact. And this change will help to transform health care delivery at all levels.

Agencies such as the American Heart Association, American Lung Association, Multiple Sclerosis Society, Arthritis Association, Diabetes Association, and American Cancer Society can explore the possibility of collaborating with each other in establishing a single, shared wellness program. Imagine the cost of a really powerful wellness and health promotion program for your clients. Yes, it is overwhelming and expensive to pursue. Now, divide the cost by ten or twelve collaborating agencies. Suddenly the impossible seems doable. Use the regional United Way to coordinate the planning and implementation of the program. This "new" way of thinking and providing service may be difficult because it is unfamiliar. But picture the community you will be living in when the change is under way.

The Mechanisms of Self-Healing: Physiology and Energetics

Most people find it valuable to know the reasons for using the self-healing and health enhancement methods. The medicine within is a very real resource with both biological and energetic features. The following discussion provides a slightly more detailed exploration of these features. For those who are learning and practicing self-healing, this knowledge builds faith. For those who are teaching or planning programs, this information helps to substantiate your proposals. Most of the physiological mechanisms triggered by the health enhancement methods are discussed in standard physiology texts (Guyton, 1995).

In conventional forms of Western exercise, the body mobilizes the best of its internal resources but then expends them fueling hungry muscles in vigorous activity. In the self-healing and health enhancement practices, the same tremendous buildup of internal resources occurs. The difference is, however, that these potent inner resources are then conserved. This becomes the medicine within. This healing resource is circulated and even

stored to sustain the strength and harmony of the dynamic interaction of tissues, organs, and glands.

In the vigorous Western practices it is not unusual for the
body to have to cross outside of its zone of comfort and safety.
One way to describe this is to say that the body crosses its
"anaerobic threshold." The general activities of health maintenance and self-healing are fueled by oxygen in the human system.
This is an "aerobic" process, meaning "with oxygen." When
under stress the body pushes the limits of its abilities; the system
needs more oxygen than it is able to process. The system transits
from healthy aerobic activity to unhealthy anaerobic activity,
meaning "lacking oxygen." The transition point is the "anaerobic
threshold."

There is a certain wisdom built into the human system. When
there is not enough oxygen, the system chooses which functions
to fuel with oxygen and which to starve, based purely on which
ones it needs to survive. It is unfortunate that the system's wisdom doesn't help us choose to stop the exercise so that it can restore its oxygen balance. But even if our inner wisdom does send
those signals, they are usually overridden by the desire to be buff,
be beautiful, or escape a dangerous threat. It is possible to operate in the anaerobic zone for brief periods. For people who are
healthy, this is not really a major problem. However, for those
who are unwell or out of balance, it can be devastating.

Numerous diseases are accelerated in the anaerobic state.
The immune system, frequently compromised in people with
health disorders, is particularly disabled by lengthy periods of
exercise that is too vigorous. One study, "Effect of Acute Exercise on Natural Killer Cell Activity in Trained and Sedentary
Human Subjects," published in the *Journal of Clinical Immunology* (Brahmi, 1985) found that it took hours for the immune system to rehabilitate when subjects pushed into the anaerobic zone
for even a few minutes. This study and numerous others also
found, in contrast, that mild fitness practices increase immune
system capacity.

Another unique point that differentiates the two kinds of fitness practices is that the mild self-healing type methods are all
done in a purposeful state of relaxation. Both Yoga from India

and Qigong from China are often called moving meditation. The interaction of deep relaxation with gentle exercise creates a special biological state that has a profound effect on the natural self-healing and health enhancement mechanisms operating within the human system.

Among the many research findings that confirm the value of the self-healing methods, one of my favorites was reported during a panel discussion at one of the major conferences on alternative and complementary medicine in Washington, D.C. Dr. Dean Ornish explained that neither age nor severity of disease was the most significant factor in predicting who would recover from heart disease (Gould, Ornish, 1995). The most important factor was the amount of change a person made in his or her life.

Dr. Ornish's research demonstrated that removal of plaque from arteries was not the only method for reducing pain and reducing the risk of death from heart disease. The plaque reduction has a definite benefit but requires time. Stress reduction and relaxation have an immediate benefit, because relaxation expands the blood vessels, reduces pressure in the circulatory system, and opens circulatory potential in blocked areas.

Regarding the economic benefit of this physiological concept, he pointed to two heart transplant cases who were on the waiting list for organ donations. After entering Dr. Ornish's self-healing program both were spared the transplant procedure. The average cost of a heart transplant is $300,000, so these two cases saved $600,000. Dr. Ornish speculated that just eliminating 10 percent of heart transplants would save approximately $10 million per year.

To keep this physiology section brief and usable, I will review in a condensed way the physiological mechanisms triggered by each of the four essential self-healing methods.

Gentle Movement

The gentle movement methods accelerate cell metabolism, which causes increased circulation of oxygen and nutrition in the blood. They gently build muscle strength, enhance balance, increase oxygen demand without spending it on muscle activity, and accelerate propulsion of lymphatic fluid, which circulates immune cells and eliminates metabolic by-products (waste, toxins) from the tissues.

Self-Massage

Self-applied massage sends reflex neurological impulses through the brain and spinal cord to organs and glands. It accelerates lymphatic circulation of immune cells and the elimination of metabolic by-products and waste from the tissue spaces. It circulates the blood. Self-massage soothes the sympathetic aspect of the autonomic nervous system, which controls the function of the organs. This produces a restorative neurotransmitter profile that includes sufficient quantities of healing chemicals such as endorphins, serotonin, and dopamine and reduced amounts of adrenaline and reduces brain-wave frequencies to the slower alpha range.

Breath Practice

The regulation of the breath shifts the nervous system toward the relaxed state, and this in turn shifts the neurotransmitter profile dramatically. It expands the blood vessels, reducing blood pressure and assisting the penetration of nutrients and oxygen deep into the capillary system; deep breaths propel the lymph fluid more dynamically than any other mechanism, which circulates immune cells and drives metabolic by-products and waste into the elimination system.

Meditation

Deep relaxation and meditation balance the parasympathetic and sympathetic aspects of the autonomic nervous system. When these two aspects are properly in balance, the state is called homeostasis. When they are out of balance, generally to the sympathetic side (fight or flight), adrenaline-based chemistry causes exhaustion and the reduction of immune system efficiency. When in balance the body chemistry is more choline based. This shifts the neurotransmitter profile to the restorative mode, which potentiates and directs immune cell activity. The brain-wave frequency shifts toward the alpha or even theta level, and the capacity of the microcirculatory system (capillaries) expands.

Energetics

The Chinese have always explained the internal power of healing in terms of Qi (Chi). They believe that the complementary energies of the earth (yin) and heaven (yang) meet within living bodies of animals, plants, and humans. This is the "original cause" of the harmonious interaction of energies known as life or vitality. The health enhancement and self-healing practices of the Chinese, called Qigong, circulate and harmonize these vital energies to maintain health and cure disease.

In India a similar belief declares that universal energies, known as Prana, circulate within the human system to sustain life and health. The practice of Yoga, the health enhancement and self-healing system of India, fosters the optimal activity of these vital energies.

Recent research in the Western sciences has begun to confirm that energy does flow within the human system. One innovative researcher, B. E. W. Nordenstrom in Sweden, has mapped the energy circulation within the human system (Nordenstrom, 1983). He calls this energy circulatory system the "vascular-interstitial closed circuitry." This is very similar to the Chinese system of energy channels called *jing luo* and the Indian system of *nadis*. Nordenstrom's name for the channels is "preferential ion conductance pathways."

The Qi, it is speculated, can mean many forms of energy from bioelectrical and magnetic to light (photons) to other subtle energies, including quantum states. Numerous organizations and institutions, including the Qigong Institute, the Institute of Noetic Sciences, the International Society for the Study of Subtle Energy and Energy Medicine, and the International Society of Life Information Science, are exploring the energetic basis of health and healing.

The physiological explanations just presented, which Western science prefers for describing the benefits of the health enhancement and self-healing methods, do not diminish the relevance of the Asian concept of energies. The two systems, one wavelike and energy based and the other substantial and materially based, are completely complementary.

An in-depth exploration of the physiological and energetic mechanisms triggered by the self-healing methods may be found in my book *The Most Profound Medicine* (Jahnke, 1990).

PHASES: A Quality-of-Life Improvement Program

I have referred to the PHASES program frequently. The acronym stands for Personal Health Action Strategies and Evaluation System. It is a simple concept. Ask yourself the following two questions about each of the areas listed here:

Question 1: Where am I now regarding this aspect of my life?
Question 2: Where would I prefer to be regarding this aspect of my life?

1 Diet and nutrition
2 Exercise and fitness
3 Stress mastery
4 Relationships and family issues
5 Work and career
6 Personal finance
7 Self-esteem
8 Play and creativity
9 Health self-care
10 Spiritual fulfillment

This process is called "self-inquiry." The gap between where you are currently and where you wish to be is the "area of improvement." The PHASES program is designed to support people in moving from where they are to where they wish to be in gradual steps or phases. In other words, you will not improve all at once but will be in the process of gradual and continuous improvement.

When you engage in this process with others, it accelerates the effect. Support, learning, accountability, and the benefits of testimonials are all supercharged by human interaction. The PHASES program is a sister to the self-healing and health enhancement methods. Look for opportunities to interact with others about their process of personal improvement through friendly communication before or after your practice sessions.

The Seven Steps of the PHASES Program

There are seven steps to the PHASES program that people can use to improve their health, either individually or in groups.

1 Self-inquiry—assessment phase
2 Evaluation and discussion of findings—exploration phase
3 Establishment of goals in several areas of improvement—planning phase
4 Personal implementation—action phase
5 Support and accountability—support and learning phase
6 Reevaluation (another round of self-inquiry)—reevaluation phase
7 Course correction—redesign phase

We have found that a group of average people can carry out a PHASES support and study group, just as a friendly activity. Using the library or the Internet as resources, a group of purposeful and inquiring people can learn a lot and have fun with the PHASES process.

Herbs, Homeopathy, and Nutrition

The effects of the methods that we have just learned can be amplified with the use of herbs. The combination of herbal formulas with the self-healing and health enhancement methods is a powerful way to enrich the medicine within. It is typical in China for people to consider herbal formulas as a key self-healing and empowerment strategy.

Here are a couple of cautions, guidelines, and suggestions.

○ Always use herbs that are considered to be nutritional and tonic. Herbs that are powerfully medicinal are actually drugs. Mahuang, poke root, lobelia, rhubarb, and cascara sagrada are a few herbs that you should never use without consulting an expert herbalist. Even with expert advice, never use these herbs unless they are in a combination that includes some tonic herbs as well.
○ Never (or at most rarely) use single herbs. Tonic and restorative herbs are always used in combinations that include at least four separate herbs. Some of the classic Chinese longevity tonics have

⌟ twenty to thirty herbs in them. Ginseng, for example, is available as a single herb, but its most effective use is in a formula with other herbs.

○ Use tonic herbal formulas preventively while you are well to stay well. These herbs are the easiest to learn to use because they require no diagnosis. They nourish and strengthen the system.

○ When you are not well, use tonics to enhance health and complement medical treatment. Western medicines generally do not cure disease by enhancing health. Tonic formulas that improve general health are excellent as complements to medical treatment (including radiation and chemotherapy) and can help to rehabilitate your vitality following medical treatment.

There are rich traditions for the use of tonic herbs in every ancient culture—China, India, Africa, Europe, and the Americas. All original cultures had three modalities of medicine and healing: herbs, massage, and the self-healing methods. When you begin to grasp the use of herbal tonics, you will have tapped into one of our most profound healing resources. Ancient, secret longevity formulas are always intended to be used in conjunction with daily practice of self-healing and health enhancement methods.

Homeopathy, while not developed by the Chinese, is completely consistent with the traditional theories of Chinese medicine. The basis of homeopathy is "vital force," which is identical to the Chinese concept of Qi (Chi). Homeopathy is sometimes preferable to herbs. It is less expensive. It is very mild yet is often dramatically effective. Because homeopathy was developed in the Western world, it is sometimes easier for people, including physicians, to embrace. Knowledge of homeopathy can eliminate unnecessary doctor visits and save money. In conjunction with the self-applied health enhancement methods and appropriate medical care, homeopathy is a powerful self-care tool.

Every family should be familiar with just a few remedies: arnica, rhus tox, bryonia, ruta, hypericum, nux vomica, gelsemium, apis, ignatia, and oscillococcinum—all in low potency.

Herbs and homeopathy are really potent and concentrated healing resources that come from the same source as food. A nutritional diet from healthful sources should always be the foundation of healthy living, self-care, and self-healing.

Bibliography and Suggested Reading

Books

The books preceded by ** are cited in the text.

Beinfield, Harriet, and Efram Korngold. *Between Heaven and Earth: A Guide to Chinese Medicine.* New York: Ballantine Books, 1992.

** Benson, Herbert, M.D. *Timeless Healing: The Power and Biology of Belief.* New York: Simon & Schuster, 1996.

** ———. *The Relaxation Response.* New York: Avon Books, 1975.

Bohm, David. *Wholeness and the Implicate Order.* New York: Routledge, 1996.

———. *The Undivided Universe.* New York: Routledge, 1995.

Borysenko, Joan. *Fire in the Soul: A New Psychology of Spiritual Optimism.* New York: Warner Books, 1994.

———. *Minding the Body, Mending the Mind.* New York: Bantam Doubleday Dell, 1993.

Cannon, Walter. *The Way of an Investigator.* New York: W. W. Norton, 1945.

Capra, Fritjof. *The Web of Life: A New Scientific Understanding of Living Systems.* New York: Anchor Books, 1996.

———. *The Tao of Physics: An Exploration of the Parallels Between Modern Physics and Eastern Mysticism.* Boston: Shambhala, 1991.

———. *The Turning Point: Science, Society, and the Rising Culture.* New York: Bantam Doubleday Dell, 1988.

** Chan, Luke. *101 Miracles of Natural Healing.* Cincinnati, OH: Benefactor Press, 1996.

Chopra, Deepak, M.D. *Ageless Body, Timeless Mind: The Quantum Alternative to Growing Old.* New York: Harmony Books, 1993.

———. *Quantum Healing: Exploring the Frontiers of Mind-Body Medicine.* New York: Bantam Doubleday Dell, 1990.

Cohen, Kenneth. *The Way of Chi Kung: The Art and Science of Chinese Energy Healing.* New York: Ballantine, 1997.

Cousins, Norman. *Head First: The Biology of Hope and the Healing Power of the Human Spirit.* New York: Penguin, 1990.

** ———. *Human Options.* New York: Berkley, 1981.

———. *Anatomy of an Illness As Perceived by the Patient: Reflections on Healing and Regeneration.* New York: W. W. Norton, 1979.

Dossey, Larry, M.D. *Prayer Is Good Medicine: How to Reap the Healing Benefits of Prayer.* San Francisco: HarperSanFrancisco, 1996.

———. *Healing Words: The Power of Prayer and the Practice of Medicine.* San Francisco: HarperSanFrancisco, 1995.

** ———. *Recovering the Soul: A Scientific and Spiritual Approach.* New York: Bantam Doubleday Dell, 1989.

———. *Space, Time and Medicine.* Boulder, CO: Shambhala, 1982.

Ferguson, Tom. *Health Online: How to Find Health Information, Support Groups, and Self-Help Communities in Cyberspace.* Boston: Addison-Wesley, 1996.

** Goldberg, Burton. *Alternative Medicine: The Definitive Guide.* Puyallup, WA: Future Medicine Publishing, 1993.

** Green, E., and A. Green. *Beyond Biofeedback.* New York: Delacourte Press, 1977.

** Guyton, Arthur C. *Textbook of Medical Physiology.* Philadelphia: Harcourt Brace Jovanovich, 1995.

** Jahnke, Roger. *Awakening and Mastering the Medicine Within* (instructional video). Santa Barbara: Health Action Publishing, 1995.

** ———. *The Most Profound Medicine.* Santa Barbara: Health Action Publishing, 1990.

Kaptchuk, Ted. *The Web That Has No Weaver: Understanding Chinese Medicine.* New York: Congdon & Weed, 1984.

** Mathews, D. A., D. B. Larson, and C. P. Barry. *The Faith Factor: An Annotated Bibliography of Clinical Research on Spiritual Subjects.* Vol. 1. Templeton Foundation, 1993.

McGarey, Gladys. *The Physician Within.* Deerfield Beach, CA: Health Communications, 1997.

McGarey, William. *In Search of Healing: Whole-Body Healing Through the Mind-Body-Spirit Connection.* Walpole, NH: Perigee Press, 1996.

McGee, Charles, and E. Poy Yew Chow. *Qigong: Miracle Healing from China.* Coeur d'Alene, ID: MediPress, 1994.

MacRitchie, James. *The Chi Kung Way.* San Francisco: HarperCollins, 1997.

————. *Chi Kung: Cultivating Personal Energy.* Dorset, England: Element Books, 1993.

** Miller, Carolyn. *Creating Miracles: Understanding the Experience of Divine Intervention.* Tiburon, CA: H. J. Kramer, 1995.

** Nordenstrom, B. E. W. *Biologically Closed Circuits: Clinical, Experimental and Theoretical Evidence for an Additional Circulatory System.* Stockholm, Sweden: Nordic Medical Publications, 1983.

Northrup, Christiane. *Women's Bodies, Women's Wisdom: Creating Physical and Emotional Health and Healing.* New York: Bantam Doubleday Dell,1994.

** O'Regan, Brendan, and Caryl Hirshberg. *Spontaneous Remission: An Annotated Bibliography.* San Francisco: Institute of Noetic Sciences Press, 1995.

** Owen, R. *Qualitative Research: Early Years.* Salem, OR: Grayhaven Books, 1988.

Ornish, Dean. *Dr. Dean Ornish's Program for Reversing Heart Disease.* New York: Random House, 1990.

Pert, Candace. *Molecules of Emotion.* New York: Scribners, 1997.

Sancier, Kenneth. *Qigong Database.* Palo Alto: Qigong Institute, 1996.

** Selye, Hans. *The Stress of Life.* New York: McGraw-Hill, 1978.

Shealy, Norman. *The Complete Family Guide to Alternative Medicine: An Illustrated Encyclopedia of Natural Healing.* Dorset, England: Element Books, 1996.

————. *Miracles Do Happen: A Physician's Experience with Alternative Medicine.* Rockport, MA: Element Books, 1996.

Siegel, Bernie, M.D. *Love, Medicine and Miracles: Lessons Learned About Self-Healing from a Surgeon's Experience with Exceptional Patients.* New York: HarperCollins, 1990.

————. *Peace, Love and Healing—Bodymind Communication and the Path to Self-Healing: An Exploration.* New York: HarperCollins, 1990.

Siou, Lily. Ch'i Kung: *The Art of Mastering the Unseen Life Force.* Honolulu: Tai Hsuan Press, 1973.

** Spiegel, David. *Living Beyond Limits.* New York: Fawcett Columbine Press, 1993.

————. *Natural Health, Natural Medicine: A Comprehensive Manual for Wellness and Self-Care.* New York: Houghton Mifflin Co., 1995.

————. *Spontaneous Healing: How to Discover and Enhance Your Body's Natural Ability to Maintain and Heal Itself.* New York: Knopf, 1995.

** Zohar, Danah, and Ian Marshall. *The Quantum Society: Mind, Physics and a New Social Vision.* New York: William Morrow, 1994.

Journal Articles

The articles preceded by ** are cited in the text.

** Bellert, J. L. "Humor. A Therapeutic Approach in Oncology Nursing." *Cancer Nurse* 12 (2):65–70, 1989.

** Berk, L. S., S. A. Tan, W. F. Fry, B. J. Napier, J. W. Lee, R. W. Hubbard, J. E. Lewis, and W. C. Eby. "Neuroendocrine and Stress Hormone Changes During Mirthful Laughter." *American Journal of Medical Science* 298 (6):390–96, Dec. 1989.

** Berkman, L. F., and S. L. Syme. "Social Networks, Host Resistance, and Mortality: A Nine-Year Follow-Up Study of Alameda County Residents." *American Journal of Epidemiology* 109 (2):186–204, Feb. 1979.

** Bernstein, L., B. E. Henderson, R. Hanisch, J. Sullivan-Halley, and R. K. Ross. "Physical Exercise and Reduced Risk of Breast Cancer in Young Women." *Journal of the National Cancer Institute* 86 (18):1403–8, Sept. 1994.

Blair, S. N., J. B. Kampert, H. W. Kohl III, C. E. Barlow, C. A. Macera, R. S. Paffenbarger, Jr., and L. W. Gibbons. "Influences of Cardiorespiratory Fitness and Other Precursors on Cardiovascular Disease and All-Cause Mortality in Men and Women." *JAMA* 276 (3):205–10, July 17, 1996.

Blair, S. N., H. W. Kohl III, C. E. Barlow, R. S. Paffenbarger, Jr., L. W. Gibbons, and C. A. Macera. "Changes in Physical Fitness and All-Cause Mortality: A Prospective Study of Healthy and Unhealthy Men." *JAMA* 273 (14):1093–98, Apr. 12, 1995.

p. 33 ** Blair, S. N., H. W. Kohl III, R. S. Paffenbarger, Jr., D. G. Clark, K. H. Cooper, L. W. Gibbons, and H. W. Kohl. "Physical Fitness and All-Cause Mortality: A Prospective Study of Healthy Men and Women." *JAMA* 262 (17):2395–401, Nov. 3, 1989.

** Brahmi, Z., J. E. Thomas, M. Park, and I. R. Dowdeswell. "The Effect of Acute Exercise on Natural Killer-Cell Activity of Trained and Sedentary Human Subjects." *Journal of Clinical Immunology* 5 (5):321–28, Sept. 1985.

** Byrd, R. C. "Positive Therapeutic Effects of Intercessory Prayer in a Coronary Care Unit Population." *Southern Medical Journal* 81 (7): 826–29, July 1988.

** Department of Health and Human Services. *Surgeon General's Report on Physical Activity and Health.* Washington, DC, 1996.

** ———. *Healthy People 2000: National Health Promotion and Disease Prevention Objectives.* Washington, DC, Publication Number (PHS) 91-50213, 1991.

** Dillbeck, M. C. "Test of a Field of Consciousness and Social Change." *Social Indicators Research* 22: 399–418, 1990.

** Fries, J. F., C. E. Koop, C. E. Beadle, P. P. Cooper, M. J. England, R. F. Greaves, J. J. Sokolov, and D. Wright. "Reducing Health Care Costs by Reducing the Need and Demand for Medical Services." The Health Project Consortium. *New England Journal of Medicine* 329 (5):321–25, July 29, 1993.

** Gold, P. W., M. A. Kling, I. Khan, J. R. Calabrese, K. Kalogeras, R. M. Post, P. C. Avgerinos, D. L. Loriaux, and G. P. Chrousos. "Corticotropin Releasing Hormone: Relevance to Normal Physiology and to the Pathophysiology and Differential Diagnosis of Hypercortisolism and Adrenal Insufficiency." *Advanced Biochemistry and Psychopharmacology* 43: 183–200, 1987.

** Goodwin, J. S., W. C. Hunt, C. R. Key, and J. M. Samet. "The Effect of Martital Status on Stage, Treatment and Survival of Cancer Patients." *JAMA* 258: 3125–30, 1987.

** Gould, K. L., D. Ornish, L. Scherwitz, S. Brown, R. P. Edens, M. J. Hess, N. Mullani, L. Bolomey, F. Dobbs, W. T. Armstrong, et al. "Changes in Myocardial Perfusion Abnormalities by Positron Emissiontomography After Long-Term, Intense Risk Factor Modification." *JAMA* 274 (11):894–901, Sept. 20, 1995.

** Grady, K. L., A. Jalowiec, C. White-Williams, R. Pifarre, J. K. Kirklin, R. C. Bourge, and M. R. Costanzo. "Predictors of Quality of Life in Patients with Advanced Heart Failure Awaiting Transplantation." *Journal of Heart and Lung Transplant* 14 (1, Pt.1): 2–10, Jan.–Feb. 1995.

** Jahnke, R. "Qigong: Awakening and Mastering the Profound Medicine Within." *American Journal of Acupuncture* 17 (2): 139–51, 1989.

** Levin, J. S. "Religion and Health." *Social Science and Medicine* 38:
1475–82, 1994.

** Lewis, P. H., and K. A. Brykczynski. "Practical Knowledge and
Competencies of the Healing Role of the Nurse Practitioner."
Journal of the American Academy of Nurse Practitioners 6
(5):207–13, May 1994.

** Oleson, T., and W. Flocco. "Randomized Controlled Study of Premenstrual Syndrome Treated with Ear, Hand, and Foot Reflexology." *Journal of Obstetrics and Gynecology* 82: 906–911, 1993.

** Orme-Johnson, D. W., and C. N. Alexander. "International Peace
Project in the Middle East: The Effect of the Maharishi Technology on the Unified Field." *Journal of Conflict Resolution* 32:
776–812, 1988.

** Ornish D., L. W. Scherwitz, R. S. Doody, D. Kesten, S. M.
McLanahan, S. E. Brown, E. DePuey, R. Sonnemaker, C. Haynes,
J. Lester, G. K. McAllister, R. J. Hall, J. A. Burdine, and A. M.
Gotto, Jr. "Effects of Stress Management Training and Dietary
Changes in Treating Ischemic Heart Disease." *JAMA* 249
(1):54–59, Jan. 7, 1983.

** Oxman, T .E., D. H. Freeman, and E.D. Manheimer. "Lack of
Social Participation or Religious Strength and Comfort as Risk
Factors for Death After Cardiac Surgery." *Psychosomatic Medicine*
57: 5–15, 1995.

** Pang, HeMing. "A Summary of Zhineng Qigong's Healing Effects
on Chronic Diseases." The Zhineng Hospital and Training Center,
1991.

** Pert, C. B., M. R. Ruff, R. J. Weber, and M. Herkenham. "Neuropeptides and Their Receptors: A Psychosomatic Network." *The
Journal of Immunology* 135 (2): 820–26, 1985.

** Pressman, P., J. S. Lyons, and J. J. Strain. "Religious Belief, Depression, and Ambulation Status in Elderly Women with Broken
Hips." *American Journal of Psychiatry* 147: 758–60, 1990.

** Roberts, Alan. "The Powerful Placebo Revisited." *Body/Mind Journal* 1 (1): 35–45, 1995.

** Salber, E. J., W. L. Beery, and E. J. Jackson. "The Role of the
Health Facilitator in Community Health Education." *Journal of
Community Health,* 2 (1):5–20, fall 1976.

** Spiegel, D., J. R. Bloom, et al. "Effect of Psychosocial Treatment on Survival of Patients with Metastatic Breast Cancer." *Lancet* 2: 888–91, 1989.

World Health Organization. *Health for All by Year 2000: Resolution of the Thirtieth World Health Assembly of the World Health Organization.* Geneva, Switzerland, 1977.

Resources

As you bring the ideas and then the methods for health enhancement and self-healing into your life, you will probably want to learn more, network with others, find a community practice session, be a mentor for friends, family, and co-workers, or lead a practice session yourself. A new wave of health enhancement and self-healing activities is expanding through hospitals, clinics, corporations, and communities in the Americas and Europe to link up with the ancient traditions of Yoga, Qigong (Chi Kung), and Taiji (Tai Chi) from China and India.

Self-Applied Health Enhancement Methods (SAHEM), Qigong, and Tai Chi: Workshops and Trainings

- Workshops and lectures
- Trainings for teachers, mentors, and health professionals
- Wellness and health promotion programs
- Healing journeys to China and Hawaii

The PHASES Program

- Computer software for self-inquiry
- Training for health care professionals
- Workshops for agencies and communities

Other Materials Available from Dr. Roger Jahnke and Health Action

- *The Healer Within* (video)
- *Awakening and Mastering the Medicine Within* (video)
- *The Most Profound Medicine* (book)
- *The Self-Applied Health Enhancement Methods* (book)
- *The PHASES Training Manual* (book)
- *Disease as Evolution* (audiotape)

   ○ *Deep Relaxation and Profound Self-Healing* (audio tape)
   ○ *Momentary Reminder Chime* (chime and instruction booklet)

Internet Resources

HealthWorld Online (Web addresses: www.healthy.net;
www.healthy.net/qigong; www.healthy.net/healerwithin)
Integral Health Network (Web addresses: www.wellness.com;
www.wellness.com/healthaction)
   These sites include:

○ "Directories" of practitioners, mentors, instructors, and practice
   locations
○ "Libraries" of information and practice instruction
○ "Forums" for interaction and discussion with like-minded practitioners of the self-healing and health enhancement arts

To receive information on the resources listed above, to order
study and practice materials, or to reach Roger Jahnke, Health
Action, and the Institute for Self-Initiated Healing, please call
1–800–824–4325. Or write to Health Action, 243 Pebble Beach,
Santa Barbara, CA 93117.

Index